the facts

Borderline personality disorder

ROY KRAWITZ
Consultant Psychiatrist
Waikato District Health Board, and
Honorary Clinical Senior Lecturer
Auckland University
New Zealand

WENDY JACKSON
Freelance Health Auditor, Quality Manager,
Consumer Advisor, and a Person who has Recovered from
Borderline Personality Disorder
Auckland, New Zealand

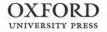

OXFORD
UNIVERSITY PRESS

OXFORD

UNIVERSITY PRESS

Great Clarendon Street, Oxford OX2 6DP

Oxford University Press is a department of the University of Oxford.
It furthers the University's objective of excellence in research, scholarship,
and education by publishing worldwide in

Oxford New York

Auckland Cape Town Dar es Salaam Hong Kong Karachi
Kuala Lumpur Madrid Melbourne Mexico City Nairobi
New Delhi Shanghai Taipei Toronto

With offices in

Argentina Austria Brazil Chile Czech Republic France Greece
Guatemala Hungary Italy Japan Poland Portugal Singapore
South Korea Switzerland Thailand Turkey Ukraine Vietnam

Oxford is a registered trade mark of Oxford University Press
in the UK and in certain other countries

Published in the United States
by Oxford University Press Inc., New York

British Library Cataloguing in Publication Data

Data available

Library of Congress Cataloguing in Publication Data

Data available

ISBN 978-0-19-920296-6 (Pbk.)

2

Typeset in Plantin
by Cepha Imaging Pvt. Ltd., Bangalore, India
Printed in Great Britain
on acid-free paper by
Clays Ltd., Bungay, Suffolk

Contents

Section 1
Borderline personality disorder information

Section 2
Recovery frameworks

Section 3
Recovery specifics

Essential notes before reading this book

This book is intended to be read in the context of receiving qualified professional help and should not be used for stand alone self-diagnosis or self-treatment. Readers are urged to seek out appropriate qualified professional help. While this book may contribute to your recovery, it is not a substitute for professional treatment.

If you are in distress please make contact with an appropriate mental health professional. If you are in danger of self-harm, please seek out professional assistance. If you have thoughts of ending your life, immediately call your therapist, doctor, emergency service, or hospital. These professionals are trained to help you in a crisis.

Foreword

Foreword by Dixianne Penney, Dr.P.H and Kiera Van Gelder, MFA

Dixianne Penney, Dr.P.H.
Co-founder and Executive Vice President, National Education Alliance for Borderline Personality Disorder, Inc. - non-profit organization that raises public awareness, provides education, and promotes research on borderline personality disorder.

Research Scientist, Center to Study Recovery in Social Contexts, Nathan Kline Institute for Psychiatric Research.

Kiera Van Gelder, MFA
Founder and Executive Director, Middle Path, Inc. - consumer organization dedicated to the advocacy, support, and education of those affected by BPD.

If you are someone currently receiving treatment or if you are thinking about seeking treatment for borderline personality disorder (BPD) then *Borderline Personality Disorder: the facts* by Roy Krawitz and Wendy Jackson needs to be on your shelf, in a handy spot.

As an informational and how-to-do-it book (a "toolbox") about how to recover from BPD, it is indispensable in many ways. The material, synthesized from the most recent scientific research on BPD and practical experience, is presented step-by-step, and can be read cover-to-cover, or used as a reference manual for different challenges faced along the path of recovery.

The book is a joint venture of a person who has recovered from BPD and her collaborator, a clinician with many years of experience. As people who have personally witnessed and experienced BPD and the transformative process of recovery, Krawitz and Jackson provide a unique beacon for anyone searching for a way out of the darkness in which BPD has so long been mired.

The combined voices of a person recovered from BPD and a BPD clinician made us feel as if we were participating in a personalized workshop with two extraordinary leaders available 24/7 at our own convenience, any time we wish to pluck the book from shelf or bedside table.

The format of the book with its chapter summaries, clear sub-headings, and personal, boxed commentaries from Wendy invites the reader in. With every suggestion there is a specific example. In addition, complementing the concrete, bringing depth to the practical illustrations, there are perceptively drawn metaphors that are crucial because they clinch the understanding of points made. For example, the authors describe the condition of BPD as like experiencing a "life that constantly feels as if you are being romantically dumped except that you are likely to feel that way over many years."

Krawitz and Jackson's writing on BPD is clear and direct, and more than any other book we know, is written specifically for the person with BPD. The use of every day language that speaks directly to the person with BPD is no indication of superficiality, or subject matter glossed over, or stones left unturned. To the contrary! *The Facts* succeeds at being both in-depth and accessible.

This practical approach, unusual in the field of BPD literature, equally emphasizes the distinct needs of every individual. "The pathway to developing the disorder will be unique for you" and therefore *you* will be a key player in your recovery. Informed choice-making is a critical component of receiving appropriate services, at all levels of recovery, and *The Facts* provides a wealth of information that empowers individuals to find the right help and to utilize it effectively.

Another key ingredient to recovery, and one often missing in the discussion of borderline personality disorder, is hope. Without hope, even the most useful tools can seem out of reach. For this reason *Borderline Personality Disorder: the facts* offers people with BPD, treatment providers, family members and all others affected by BPD, a tremendous and potentially life-changing gift.

Their message comes through over and over again: **People can and do recover from borderline personality disorder**. This fact is rightfully underscored in every section.

The authors' personal experience with successful treatment and recovery presages a new era in BPD literature, as does their collaboration on the book, a landmark achievement in a field where the diagnosis has often signified a person's unwillingness to engage in treatment. Recovery, Krawitz and Jackson show us, is real. But they are also honest and respectful about the hard work and difficulties faced along the way, and they urge us to give change a chance.

We are particularly impressed by Roy and Wendy's attention to those for whom the phrase BPD has been a block to receiving help for the pain they are in. Toss it, they counsel, if it gets in your way. "Use it if it helps you." They are equally attentive to those who may have been the recipients of a long line of diagnoses, none really seeming to fit: "If you have been in the mental health system for a long time and have only recently been given a BPD diagnosis, do not despair, this could represent a major turning point in your recovery."

Wise counsel also from Wendy and Roy that your recovery is not a race, and not to set yourself up as if you were entering Olympic trials where winners continue and losers drop out; support for times of rest if need be, a "pacing" as the writers term it, decided by *you*, in charge and responsible for your life and your therapeutic journey and recovery.

We are honored to be writing this foreword to *The Facts*. We share a similar, although more recent, partnership, in that we also collaborate on projects of advocacy, training, teaching and writing about BPD. Kiera, a recipient of services, who considers herself a 'work in progress' is an artist, writer and educator who founded Middle Path, a United States-based consumer organization dedicated to the advocacy, support and education of those affected by BPD. Dixie, a family member of long-standing whose family can still find itself occasionally on a challenging roller coaster wondering if the brakes will work, is a Co-founder and Executive Vice President of the National Education Alliance for Borderline Personality Disorder, Inc., also U.S.-based, a non-profit organization that raises public awareness, provides education, promotes research on borderline personality disorder, and enhances the quality of life of those affected by this serious mental illness. Dixie has spent her 30-year professional career in both the public and private sectors in mental health administration.

In writing this foreword, we have learned so much from Wendy and Roy. With this volume they herald the value and successful partnership of two experts in the field of borderline personality disorder: one who has walked the personal road of recovery and one who has the requisite professional credentials to collaborate with her, whose complementary points of view and experiences have positioned them to write a book that will stand the test of time.

Borderline Personality Disorder: the facts not only takes its place but rises to the top as a welcome addition among the few books that are really helpful to persons with BPD (Bockian et al, 2002[1]; Friedel, 2004[2]; Gunderson & Hoffman, eds., 2005[3]). We consider it to be the most down-to-earth, accessible book for people with BPD to date and one which we wholeheartedly recommend to anyone seeking the path of recovery.

Dixianne Penney, Dr.P.H. and Kiera Van Gelder, MFA

References

1. Bockian, N.R., Villagran, N.E., & Porr, V. (2002). *New Hope for People with Borderline Personality Disorder: Your Friendly, Authoritative Guide to the Latest in Traditional and Complementary Solutions*. Roseville, CA: Prima Publishing (a division of Random House).

2. Friedel, R.O. (2004) *Borderline Personality Disorder Demystified*. Marlow & Co. New York, NY.

3. Gunderson, J.G. & Hoffman, P.D. (Eds.) (2005) *Understanding and Treating Borderline Personality Disorder: A Guide for Professionals and Families*. American Psychiatric Press, Inc. Washington, DC.

Acknowledgements

We would like to express our appreciation to those people with borderline personality disorder who have shared their knowledge and experiences with us. Without you this book would not have been possible. Your knowledge and experiences of both private and public service treatment have now come full circle, being returned back to people with borderline personality disorder in the form of this book.

We wish to acknowledge those whose ideas and writings have shaped our thinking in the writing of this book. Anthony Bateman (mentalizing), Mary Ellen Copeland (consumer recovery), Marsha Linehan (DBT) and Bill Miller (human change), all brilliant people who revolutionized their respective fields. Also, those clinicians (including DiClimente, Miller S, Norcross, Prochaska), whose trans-theoretical ideas have encouraged us to respect several treatments and to search for common ground between these treatments.

Thanks to the Waikato District Health Board as an organization and specifically to Chris Harris, Eileen Hughes, Rajiv Singh, Wendy Tuck, and Carole Kennedy for believing in the rights to effective treatment for people with borderline personality disorder well ahead of the times and for providing the supportive administrative structures that have supported our work.

We would like to thank Graham Mellsop and the Waikato Clinical School, University of Auckland for their sizeable and specific support of this project.

Thank you also to the Waikato Hospital librarians (Lynda Pryor, Sharon Cornwall, Angela Broring, Carolyn Bruce, Trish Houchen, Tracy Robinson, Jenny McIvor, Kathy Ooi, Lyn Wood, Julia Gryaznova) who have over the years always been superefficient and welcoming despite the vast amount of work that we have generated for them. Without your time and energy we would not have been able to keep abreast with the knowledge required to write this book.

This book would not have been possible without the discussions we have had with our colleagues and friends. These include Nick Argyle, Jon Ballantyne, Jane Barrington, Mike Batcheler, Glenn Bradburn, Pip Bradley, Vicki Burnett, Sandy Byers Evitt, Deb Christensen, Emily Cooney, Carolyn Dewe, Sue Fitchett, John Gawith, Catherine Gilberd, Ora Guptill, Carole Kennedy, Kirsten van Kessel, Sue Robertson, Gail Robinson, Gael Rowntree, David Semp, SKIP network members, Elizabeth Simpson, Alice Stephan, Kirsten Thickpenny-Davis, Christine Watson, and Pat Wood. Thanks to Vicki Burnett, Deb Christensen, SKIP network members, and Pat Wood who have supported us during the writing of this book.

Thanks from me (Wendy) to Gail Robinson for her unfailing belief in my ability to support others with borderline personality disorder and her faith to involve me in training clinicians long before consumer trainers were considered acceptable let alone desirable. My special thanks also to the clinicians who walked my journey with me and never gave up on their belief in my ability to recover. Also, to my family (including Glenda, Claire, and Fleur). I know that parts fo my journey were as hard for you as they were for me. Thank you for doing what needed to be done, and sharing the ongoing joys of recovery with me.

Our deepest thanks to our reviewers, Kiera van Gelder and Pat Wood, who without payment gave generously of their time and energy sharing with us their vast experience and wisdom, resulting in substantial improvements in the quality of the book. A big thank you also to Dixianne Penney and Kiera Van Gelder who willingly gifted their time, energy, knowledge, and experience in writing their foreword.

We wish to express our appreciation to Oxford University Press for their interest and enthusiasm in getting this book off the ground, converting an idea into actual reality, and providing the administrative and logistical input required to bring this book to its final product.

Introduction

Welcome

Welcome—a very warm welcome. We hope that you find this book a helpful resource in maximizing your recovery and healing. In writing this book we have combined our knowledge from different experiences as person robustly recovered from borderline personality disorder (Wendy) and therapist/ psychiatrist specializing in the treatment of people with borderline personality disorder (Roy). Our relationship has always been as colleagues and never as clinician and client, and is deeply collaborative in our shared tasks of borderline personality disorder advocacy, training, and writing. We view our different perspectives and collaborative spirit as important and valuable dimensions resulting in a book we believe to be more useful than either of us could have produced alone. Much of our learning has come from people with borderline personality disorder and it gives us great satisfaction to be returning this knowledge back to where it came from—to people with the condition referred to as borderline personality disorder.

If you are put off by the term 'borderline personality disorder', you might wish immediately to read the section **'Not getting derailed by the term 'borderline personality disorder'** in this introduction.

About the book

This book is intended as an adjunct to support your therapy and not for stand alone self-diagnosis or self-treatment. **If you are not in therapy and think you might have borderline personality disorder, seek out a professional opinion**.

We have written this book assuming that you know you have borderline personality disorder or traits of the condition, are wondering whether you have the condition or traits of the condition, or someone has advised you that you have or might have the condition or traits* of the condition. We have written this book speaking directly to you as someone with the condition. If you do not have the condition yourself and/or are a professional, family member, or friend we thank you for your interest and willingness to read the book and hope that you find the book useful.

The inspiration and initial ideas for this book included Wendy's personal experience of wanting but not having a book when she needed it that was written directly for her and that was both informative and reader friendly. Further inspiration came from people-in-recovery who have asked for such a book for themselves and clinicians who told us how helpful such a book would be for clients they see.

Borderline personality disorder was once the poor cousin of mental health conditions. Scientific knowledge about treatment lagged behind knowledge of other mental health conditions. Historically, reported outcomes were poor and there was limited scientific literature about the condition. This has now thankfully changed. Clinicians began modifying and improving treatments with improved outcomes. The first scientifically robust report of effective treatment was published in 1991, with reports of effective treatment being published since then at an increasing rate. Research to date has shown that a number of different treatments can be effective in the treatment of people with borderline personality disorder. Published literature for professionals in the form of scientific papers and technical books has grown rapidly.

However, there has been a lag in information and literature for you, a person with the condition. This book aims to address this gap, providing up to date information about your condition in an easy reading informal writing style. The book deliberately has you as a person with borderline personality disorder as the most important readership—you have been at the forefront of our attention and our primary focus when we have been writing this book.

This book has been informed by research data, expert opinion, and guidelines from literature in the field. We include the latest current professional and consumer information synthesized with our personal and professional experience and presented in a deliberately informal style that is both direct and clear. Scientific references have been purposefully mostly left out to smooth the reading. The book has been appraised and reviewed by both clinicians and consumers. Wherever possible we have used everyday non-professional language; however, some words remain that require clarification. These words are noted with an *asterisk* * next to the word and listed alphabetically in the glossary at the end of the book with an explanation of meaning.

Section 1

In Section 1, we provide factual information on borderline personality disorder written specifically with you as the reader in mind.

Section 2

In Section 2, we provide information to assist you in setting up frameworks and structures for your effective treatment, recovery, and healing, including believing you can recover, getting yourself ready for change, selecting a therapist, and making the most out of the treatments that are available to you.

Section 3

In Section 3, we outline some specific strategies that you might find helpful for everyday living. A comprehensive discussion of all possible skills is beyond the scope of this book. Instead, we have selected skills that are practical and of recognized value in everyday life. Some of the specific strategies will be sufficient as written in this book while others serve to illuminate areas of fruitful discussion and exploration with your therapist.

How you can read the book

There are a number of flexible ways to read this book. The book can be read from cover to cover if you have the time and concentration. Reading this way, each Section of the book serves as a foundation for later Sections. Alternatively you can start with Section 1, Section 2, or Section 3 depending on your immediate interests.

If you feel that you have enough information on borderline personality disorder and want to move straight on to reading about what you can do, you might choose to skip Section 1 or perhaps return to it later. Some of you might find Section 1 compelling, while others might find Section 1 to be fairly dry and less engaging than Sections 2 and 3. In general, we think that for most readers the book will become increasingly engaging from Section 1, through Section 2, and then to Section 3. So, if you are reading Section 1 and find it excessively dry and hard going, you might want to switch to Sections 2 and 3. We would much prefer you did this than abandon the book before reading Sections 2 and 3. You might wish to return to aspects of Section 1, Section 2, or Section 3 as circumstances evolve.

At the beginning of each chapter is a summary of key points in the chapter. If you do not have the time or concentration to read whole chapters, you could start by reading these chapter summaries and then go back to read those chapters that most interest you. The layout of the book includes numerous headings, real life examples, and Wendy sharing her personal experiences that make for variety and ease of reading.

We encourage you to write all over the book highlighting and underlining parts that make sense to you, which can serve to focus your attention for future reading or if you wish to have a quick second or third read. Alternatively, a full second or third read may uncover new material that draws your attention.

Not getting derailed by the term 'borderline personality disorder'

The book has been written specifically for you if you are someone with the condition referred to by mental health professionals as 'borderline personality disorder'. It is important not to get derailed by the terms 'personality disorder' or 'borderline personality disorder'. Generally personality disorder refers to ongoing patterned ways of relating to oneself and the world that is ineffective, causes distress to oneself, and refers to current aspects of the person—*it is not who the person is*. We are eager at the very outset that the term 'borderline personality disorder' does not get in the way of benefits you might gain from reading this book. Some people with 'borderline personality disorder' are comfortable with the term 'borderline personality disorder', having found the term extremely helpful, others are neutral to the term, while others are uncomfortable with the term, finding it offensive and counterproductive. The term 'borderline personality disorder' has historically often been associated with putting down, negative and derogatory views of the person with the condition. One of the reasons for this was because clinicians didn't know how to treat the person with borderline personality disorder and often blamed the client for the very behaviours that brought them into treatment. Fortunately this is now changing. You will have your own experiences and thoughts about the advantages and disadvantages of diagnosing and labelling someone with any diagnosis and in particular a diagnosis of borderline personality disorder. If a diagnosis of borderline personality disorder will help you achieve your goals, then use it. If it will detract from achieving these goals then dispense with it. The name, label, or diagnosis is not nearly as important as the substance behind it and directions for treatment and solutions to your difficulties. At the end of the day what is important is that you seek out and engage actively in skilful effective treatment for the difficulties you have, working towards the goals you wish to achieve.

To get around some of these difficulties, we considered using the phrase 'people meeting diagnostic criteria for borderline personality disorder' but decided against this due to the phrase being a bit of a mouthful and rather unwieldy to use throughout the book. We have opted instead to use the shorter and more easily read phrase, 'people with borderline personality disorder'. We are mindful that shorthand terms can have the effect of diminishing the personhood of an individual; however, as we use the term 'borderline personality disorder' over 200 times in the book, we have, for ease of reading, abbreviated 'borderline personality disorder' to 'BPD', a term used by many people with borderline personality disorder to describe themselves.

We have chosen to use the term 'borderline personality disorder' as it is the most commonly agreed upon term and the language most commonly used to describe, research, and illuminate effective treatments for the condition. We encourage you to stay focused on what is behind the term and implications for effective treatment and not get derailed by some of the negative associations that you might have encountered with the term.

I am in … treatment. Can this book help support me in my treatment?

We have personally witnessed different pathways to recovery and healing and believe that this book could be useful for readers engaged in a range of different treatments.

Hope

This book is about hope—credible and realistic hope. Modern research has shown that the prognosis* for the condition is far better than we previously believed, probably due to the major treatment advances made in the last 20 years. There is now a robust research base demonstrating that treatment can be effective. We share scientific information about treatment from this research augmented by expert opinion about principles of effective recovery. Wendy's history of recovery provides hope in a manner that is personal, engaging, and alive, and both of us (Wendy and Roy) share, from our experiences, factors that we have seen to be most helpful to people with borderline personality disorder. We do not have magic or quick solutions to all of your problems. Rather, we wish to validate the severity of your distress, the challenges of change, and provide a structure to hopefully support you in your recovery. Our wish is that this book helps you in getting your life on track and then keeping your life on track. We have enjoyed writing this book and hope you enjoy reading it. We wish you the very best in your reading, recovery, and healing.

Information about the authors

Roy

Roy is a consultant psychiatrist and therapist with 25 years experience as a borderline personality disorder therapist, consultant, trainer, researcher, and scientific author. Roy has provided borderline personality disorder therapy (DBT, psychodynamic, and supportive psychotherapy) in public, private, individual, group, community, outpatient, acute, crisis, substance use, and residential mental health settings. Roy is an Honorary Clinical Senior Lecturer at Auckland University. Published scientific research includes the effectiveness of his therapy, the DBT programme he works in and his borderline personality disorder training for professionals (2500 trained). This is Roy's fourth published book on borderline personality disorder, one of which (published by Oxford University Press) has also been translated into and published in Dutch and Japanese.

Wendy

Wendy is an ex-consumer of services for people with borderline personality disorder, has been employed as a mental health promoter for a national mental health organization, and is a freelance health auditor, quality manager, and consumer advisor. Wendy has 'been there and done that' having benefited from treatment implemented across inpatient, community, and crisis services and now has a robust history of recovery from borderline personality disorder. Wendy's current role as a consumer of services for bipolar disorder, which developed four years after recovering from borderline personality disorder, ensures that she remains personally knowledgeable, abreast of, and active in the full range of current consumer issues including her role as Chair of the Northern Regional Consumer Network. In her role as consumer consultant, Wendy has been actively involved in the setting up and delivery of treatment plans, running skills training and support groups for clients with borderline personality disorder, and delivering borderline personality disorder trainings to professionals.

Roy and Wendy

Roy and Wendy collaborate in jointly providing borderline personality disorder advocacy, training for professionals, authoring articles, and of course have jointly written this book. Published research has demonstrated that their jointly provided borderline personality disorder trainings for clinicians outperformed trainings that already had evidence of effectiveness run by Roy alone.

Wendy's experience

I was treated over a 10-year period in acute, crisis, and community mental health services that were largely ineffective and was on the receiving end of some very putting down and derogatory attitudes. A major turning point occurred when I was accurately diagnosed, following which appropriate treatment was discussed and delivered, and I recovered. It is now 7 years since I met criteria for borderline personality disorder. My life was sheer hell and now is mostly satisfying and meaningful; not perfect, but certainly content and filled with a good deal of happiness and peace.

Language

Self-harm

Self-harm refers to harm deliberately inflicted upon the body usually as a means of relieving emotional distress, and can take many forms. While we do write specifically about self-harm, we have chosen not to focus on the single behaviour of self-harm or use the term 'self-harm' in the title of the book and as a way of describing the condition where criteria for the diagnosis of borderline personality disorder exist. Our view is that the use of the term 'self-harm' might have been appropriate in the past when the attitudinal response of clinicians to the term 'borderline personality disorder' was substantially negative and associated with despair and hopelessness. As this is now significantly changing we believe that focusing on 'borderline personality disorder' where applicable, while having some disadvantages, has greater advantages as it encourages attention to be given by you to many aspects of your condition that may include but also goes beyond self-harm.

Consumer, client, person-in-recovery

It is our belief that people with borderline personality disorder need to be referred to using terms chosen by themselves. In our experience these terms are usually 'client', 'consumer', or 'person-in-recovery', so these terms have been used interchangeably throughout the book. The term 'client' or 'person-in-recovery' are preferred to 'patient' as they suggest a more active role, so important for recovery from the borderline personality disorder condition. The term 'person-in-recovery' is preferred by many as the terms 'client' or 'consumer' in other contexts imply choice, which is often not the case in public mental health services or in insurance-funded treatment services. The term 'person-in-recovery' is also self-evidentially hopeful.

'Case management' (sic)

This is a term that we have avoided wherever possible as it imparts a message, albeit often unintentional, that we believe is not helpful. We believe people with borderline personality disorder should be referred to as people not 'cases' and should receive treatment rather than be 'managed'. We have used the term in four paragraphs so as to be inclusive of yourself if this is the name given to treatment that you are receiving. In these four paragraphs we have placed the term 'case management' in single quotation marks followed by (sic), which is the standard way of indicating that a term referred to is not that of the authors. The term 'case management' is well entrenched in many systems and in no way do we suggest that receiving a 'case management' approach will be unhelpful, or that the people providing 'case management' have unhelpful attitudes, merely that, in our opinion, the wording is less than ideal. An alternative term could be 'recovery co-ordinator'.

Abbreviations

BPD	Borderline personality disorder
DBT	Dialectical behaviour therapy
DSM-IV	*Diagnostic and statistical manual of mental disorders*, 4th edition

Section 1

Borderline personality disorder

Information

In Section 1, we provide factual information on borderline personality disorder written specifically with you as the reader in mind. If you feel that you have enough information on borderline personality disorder and want to move straight onto reading about what you can do, you might choose to skip Section 1 or perhaps return to it later. Some of you might find Section 1 compelling, while others might find Section 1 to be fairly dry and less engaging than Sections 2 and 3. So, if you are reading Section 1 and find it excessively hard going, you might want to switch to Sections 2 and 3. We would much prefer you did this than abandon the book before reading Sections 2 and 3. You might wish to return to aspects of Section 1 as circumstances evolve.

1

History

The term 'borderline personality disorder' was initially suggested in the 1930s by therapists as a means of identifying a group of clients who did not fit into the usual categorizations at the time. Back then, people-in-recovery were broadly categorized as either 'neurotic'*, including what we now refer to as anxiety and depressive disorders, or 'psychotic'*, including what we now refer to as bipolar disorder* and schizophrenia*. Therapists found that there was a group of clients who in many ways fitted into the 'neurotic' category except that they did not respond to the usual treatments at the time. The term 'borderline' referred to the belief at the time that this group of people were on the 'border' between neurotic and psychotic. While some people with BPD do have occasional psychotic or psychotic-like experiences, this definition of BPD being on the 'border' no longer applies; however, the term has become ingrained.

For the majority of the twentieth century, treatment outcomes for people diagnosed with BPD were generally poor. Clinicians and research scientists turned their energies and interests in other directions. In the late twentieth century, clinicians began successfully modifying and adapting their treatments, resulting in improved outcomes for people diagnosed with BPD. Professional and scientific interest in the condition soared and continues to grow. People with the condition and their families have been speaking out, which led to improved professional attitudes, funding of treatment, and funding of research into the condition.

There have been significant breakthroughs in treatment approaches, and research into understanding and improving treatments is on the increase. The first scientific evidence of effective treatment was published in 1991, representing a major turning point in the treatment of people with BPD. No longer could people be denied treatment on the basis that there was no evidence of the effectiveness of treatment. Since 1991, there have been further reports of effective treatment, with publications growing at an increased rate. The growing base of scientific evidence that treatment can be effective and improved clinician attitudes mean that clinicians are more likely nowadays to be positive and focused on providing effective treatment than in the past. People such as yourself are now either recognized or beginning to be recognized as having a disabling condition that is often extremely severe and warranting compassionate and effective treatment. People like yourself with BPD are beginning to take a rightful deserving place in mental health treatment services, alongside people with other severe disabling mental health conditions.

Professional attitudes

The term 'borderline personality disorder' has historically often been associated with negativity and derogatory, blaming, and putting down attitudes among professionals. People with the condition, families, friends, and professionals spoke out raising these problems. This consumer, family, and professional voice, increased professional interest, improved treatments, and evidence of effective treatments have all contributed to generally improved attitudes of professionals in the twenty-first century. While some clinicians continue with their unfounded negative attitudes, many more professionals now have a positive approach to people like yourself.

 Comment from Wendy

When I was doing my nursing training in the mid-1980s, I was taught that people with the diagnosis of BPD should be avoided and engaging with them could be dangerous. Thankfully things have improved greatly. I provide BPD training to mental health clinicians and am still sometimes shocked by outdated attitudes; however, I find that the vast majority of clinicians now have a compassionate and warm attitude and a desire to do their best for people with BPD.

2

How many people have borderline personality disorder?

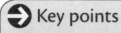 **Key points**

- Research indicates that about 0.5–2.0% of adults living in developed Western countries probably have the condition.

- Seventy-five per cent of those diagnosed are female.

- Many people have some of the features of BPD but at a level that does not significantly interfere with their lives.

Research indicates that about 0.5–2.0% of adults living in developed Western countries probably have the condition and there is subjective information that the number of people meeting criteria for BPD is increasing. There are suggestions that BPD might be far less common in other countries and cultures.

As yet unanswered questions are whether the number of people meeting criteria for BPD would be less in cultures where strong family and extended family connections remain. Some experts suggest that the movement of people to cities, increased family mobility, loss of the small village culture, and fewer family and extended family connections are all socio-cultural factors that increase the likelihood of people developing BPD. It is suggested that nuclear families do not have the same protection as the small village and extended family culture.

Seventy-five per cent of those diagnosed are female. Many authors believe males are under-represented and underdiagnosed in mental health settings and more likely to be found (but not diagnosed) in substance use centres and in the justice system. Seventy per cent of those diagnosed have a history of past sexual abuse with 46% having a history of being victims of adult violence.

Can I have a little bit of BPD?

To meet criteria for the diagnosis according to the *Diagnostic and statistical manual of mental disorders*, 4th edn (DSM-IV*), you have to have five out of a possible nine criteria. If you have three or four of the possible nine BPD features, you fall below the five features limit for having the condition and you could be said to have BPD traits* (features), if the features are enduring and causing significant life problems. Many people have some of the features of BPD but at a level that does not significantly interfere with their lives.

If you are using or abusing alcohol and/or other drugs you may well be very emotionally distressed and have features of BPD. For example, if your physiology (the workings of your physical body) is all over the place because you are taking street heroin at irregular intervals and with varying dosages, then of course you will be emotionally uneven. In this situation and other substance use situations, it is worth holding back from making the diagnosis if possible until you have stabilized your substance use. Having said this, it is very common for people with BPD to have substance use problems as well, so of course the two very often coexist side by side.

It is important to note that BPD is a diagnosis usually applied only to adults. As adolescence is a period when many BPD features occur as part of normal adolescent development, clinicians tend to prefer not to make the diagnosis in teenage years. The term 'emerging BPD' is sometimes used to describe youth who are having problems related to BPD features but who are too young to be sure that they will have the condition as they enter adulthood.

BPD often overlaps with other conditions such as depression, anxiety, substance use, eating disorders, and other psychological difficulties (see Chapter 5— 'Other problems or diagnoses found in association with BPD').

3

What is borderline personality disorder?

> **⊘ Key points**

> ◆ BPD is a recognizable real condition that deserves attention and treatment.

> ◆ BPD is a term given to a condition with a collection of features.

> ◆ To meet diagnostic criteria for BPD you will need to have five or more of the listed features in the DSM-IV criteria.

> ◆ Whether you choose to call your condition BPD or not, is not important.

> ◆ Diagnosis can serve as a guide to effective and compassionate treatment.

> ◆ Alternative names for the collection of features that we call BPD exist.

> ◆ We have adapted the formal technical diagnostic criteria used by professionals into a series of questions using common use language. If you are wondering whether you might have BPD, ask yourself the questions in Table 3.1.

BPD is a recognizable and real condition that deserves attention and treatment. People like yourself with BPD are recognized as having significant emotional pain in a number of areas including anxiety (fear, terror), sadness, depression, shame, guilt, emptiness, and loneliness.

To diagnose or not to diagnose?

In the introduction to the book we encouraged you to understand your condition and to put in place effective treatment for your condition. Whether you call your condition BPD or not, is not critical. BPD was included in the DSM-IV, the major diagnostic reference manual for professionals, as a mental health diagnosis when a group of professionals got together and decided that there were advantages in giving a name to a collection of features that they frequently encountered. Disadvantages can occur if the diagnosis is associated with negativity, pessimism, or derogatory attitudes, or with a failure to recognize the uniqueness and humanity of the person with the condition. The most important advantage is that diagnosis can serve as a guide to effective and compassionate treatment. Other advantages include sourcing education about the condition, a common language for professionals and people-in-recovery to use as a reference point to know that they are talking about the same condition, research into understanding the condition, and research into effective treatments. Increasingly people like yourself with BPD are being told about the diagnosis, assisting you in being informed, and being able to join together with your therapist as a true collaborative team working together, each with responsibilities.

Alternative names used to describe BPD

There have been explorations of alternative names for the collection of features that we call BPD. 'Complex post-traumatic stress disorder' acknowledges in the name the role of past trauma, while 'emotion regulation disorder' and 'emotional intensity disorder' highlight the central feature of heightened emotional sensitivity and reactivity.

A useful way of thinking about BPD is that of ongoing, enduring instability in many areas of life including thoughts, emotions, behaviours, and relationships. We like the term 'emotion regulation disorder', if not as a diagnostic name, as a way of understanding the condition and as a way of thinking to aid treatment and recovery. Emotion dysregulation refers to rapid shifts in emotions where we do not feel in charge, as our emotional selves take charge in a way that is unhelpful or harmful. If our problem is one of emotion dysregulation then it is obvious that solutions and treatment will include developing the skills necessary to take charge and regulate our emotions.

Features of BPD

BPD is a term given to a condition with a collection of features. Most experts in the field recognize BPD as a valid recognizable condition despite some grey areas at the edges. As a basis for initial discussion we have listed the criteria for BPD as they are listed in the DSM-IV—the major diagnostic reference manual for professionals. After this we have explored diagnosis by providing a series of questions you might ask yourself in common use language.

To meet diagnostic criteria for BPD you will need to have five or more of the listed features in the DSM-IV criteria. It is important to note that the features also need to be:

◆ pervasive: occurring in a wide range of personal and social situations

◆ enduring: long-standing, onset in adolescence or adulthood, and stable over time

◆ and lead to significant distress or impairment in functioning.

Diagnostic criteria for borderline personality disorder—DSM-IV

(*Reprinted with permission from the* Diagnostic and Statistical Manual of Mental Disorders, *Fourth Edition. Text Revision (Copyright 2000), American Psychiatric Association).*

A pervasive pattern of instability of interpersonal relationships, self-image, and affects*, and marked impulsivity beginning by early adulthood and present in a variety of contexts, as indicated by five (or more) of the following:

(1) frantic efforts to avoid real or imagined abandonment. Note: do not include suicidal or self mutilating behavior covered in Criterion 5

(2) a pattern of unstable and intense interpersonal relationships characterized by alternating between extremes of idealization and devaluation

(3) identity disturbance: markedly and persistently unstable self-image or sense of self

(4) impulsivity in at least two areas that are potentially self-damaging (e.g. spending, sex, substance abuse, reckless driving, binge eating). Note: do not include suicidal or self-mutilating behaviour covered in Criterion 5

(5) recurrent suicidal behaviour, gestures or threats, or self–mutilating behaviour.

---

(6) affective instability due to a marked reactivity of mood (e.g. intense episodic dysphoria, irritability or anxiety usually lasting a few hours and only rarely more than a few days)

(7) chronic feelings of emptiness

(8) inappropriate intense anger or difficulty controlling anger (e.g. frequent displays of temper, constant anger, recurrent physical fights)

(9) transient, stress related paranoid ideation or severe dissociative symptoms

One way of thinking about the main features of BPD is to group them into an:

◆ emotion group (highly reactive mood and emotions, unstable relationships emptiness, abandonment fears, excessive anger)

◆ impulsivity group (e.g. self-harm, substance use)

◆ identity group (emptiness, abandonment fears, unstable self-image/sense of self).

We have adapted the formal technical diagnostic criteria used by professionals, feature by feature, into a series of parallel questions using common use language. If you are wondering whether you might have BPD, ask yourself the questions shown in Table 3.1.

Table 3.1 If you are wondering whether you might have BPD, ask yourself the following questions:

1. Am I scared of rejection and abandonment, and being left all alone?
2. Are my relationships with my friends and family unstable? Do I see things as either all good or all bad; 100% right or 100% wrong?
3. Do I have trouble knowing who I am?
4. Do I impulsively do things which might damage me in some way?
5. Do I self-harm or behave in a suicidal manner?
6. Do I have mood swings that could change quickly?
7. Do I feel empty and feel I need others to fill me up and make me whole?
8. Do I get excessively angry in a manner that is to my own detriment?
9. Do I numb out (dissociate) or sometimes feel paranoid when stressed?

4

Understanding borderline personality disorder

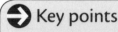 **Key points**

- It is important that diagnosis is only one part of understanding your unique personhood.

- A diagnosis alone is not enough for understanding yourself and provides insufficient information to guide treatment effectively.

- If you meet the criteria for BPD, you are likely to have had a very difficult life.

We are all much, much, much more than a diagnosis

It is important that diagnosis is only one part of understanding your unique personhood and that the diagnosis is integrated with other ways of understanding yourself. These understandings of yourself can then be used to set out a plan of treatment and active engagement in effective treatment. A diagnosis alone is insufficient for understanding yourself and provides insufficient information to guide treatment effectively by failing to identify specifically unique factors that are most important in your problems and in solutions to your problems. A diagnosis alone can also be dehumanizing.

Comment from Wendy

A diagnosis is simply a way of people, particularly professionals getting some understanding of you, to aid in planning with you, a way forward. You are not, never were, and will never be 'a borderline'—that is impossible. You may meet diagnostic criteria for BPD as a part of who you are, but you will never be 'a borderline'. Any therapist worth their salt will spend a lot of time finding out about your strengths and all the other parts of who you are to gain a balanced whole picture.

When I was diagnosed with BPD, the common language used was that I 'was' a borderline personality disorder. I hated this, emphasizing for me the sense that I was entirely damaged. Throughout the world, many of us involved in assisting change have turned language around so that now we speak of ourselves and assert our right to be spoken of as 'someone who meets diagnostic criteria for BPD or who has BPD'. This sits much better with me, as it indicates that this is just one part of what made up the person that was me.

Brief outline of causes of BPD

We discuss possible causes of BPD in detail in a later chapter but wished briefly to say enough about cause here to put into context our discussion in this chapter on understanding BPD. There are many factors that can contribute to the way that BPD can develop, including biological predisposition (factors making it more likely to develop BPD) and psychological trauma. About 15–20% of the population are thought to be born with a temperament where emotions are experienced intensely (biological predisposition). This has advantages and disadvantages and is neither good nor bad *per se* but requires understanding to make the most out of our biological make up. You may have been born feeling emotions intensely, into a caring family who did their very best, not knowing exactly how to respond to your emotional intensity. This may have left you feeling misunderstood despite the best efforts of yourself and your family, with no one to blame. Others may have had severe psychologically traumatic experiences such as childhood sexual abuse and/or physical assault. Both these situations of biological predisposition and psychological trauma could have made it difficult or impossible to develop necessary psychological skills and resulted in the behaviours that are categorized as BPD.

Making sense of all the DSM-IV diagnostic criteria together

Now, we make sense of the DSM criteria as a whole, highlighting in bold italics key phrases that are associated with the nine DSM-IV criteria listed towards the end of Chapter 4.

If you are an intense or emotionally sensitive person, as many people with BPD are, you might respond enthusiastically when things are going well and plummet when things are not going well. You are likely to be sensitive to events in the world around you (especially relationships) and also to your own self-talk, which might be quite harsh on yourself. This is likely to be associated with and result in very ***high levels of reactivity of your mood*** with rapid changes that can be extremely unsettling. Your emotions and moods might be very labile—easily go up and down in response to events with little time in an even more settled mid-range. Because your emotions are so intense, it is more challenging for you to use skilful behaviours when distressed. It is more likely therefore that your behaviour will be determined by your mood; that is, mood-dependent behaviour rather than skilful behaviour whatever your mood.

If you have BPD, you are likely to have had a difficult life either due to the difficulties of being born experiencing emotions intensely in a world not knowing how to relate to this intensity or due to childhood trauma, or a combination of the two. This could have resulted in your not having had the necessary positive opportunities to develop a robust sense of self-worth and self-esteem. If your life has been full of such experiences, you will of course be unhappy and may be depressed. Life might be hellish.

Difficulties with emotion regulation might show themselves in the present in difficulty with self-esteem and knowing who you are (***identity***) and what you believe in (values). If your emotions change rapidly and intensely, it might be hard to know your values steadily and have a stable sense of your own ***identity***. If your identity and self-esteem are linked to being with another person, then it makes sense that you will be ***anxious about being rejected and abandoned*** and wish not to be alone, to keep away feelings of ***emptiness***. Rapidly changing emotions and easily changing identity and values are likely to be associated with parallel changes in ***relationships that will be inherently unstable*** and perhaps turbulent. This may include considerable arguing and possibly break-ups and reconciliations. If you lean on other people to get by, it is quite likely that you will at times see them in a very positive and perhaps idealizing way. If these people are unable to meet your expectations then it makes sense that you will feel disappointed in them and perhaps cope with your disappointment by devaluing them and **getting very angry**. This **idealizing and devaluation** will be very hard on you and the people you are in a relationship with. There will be an ever-changing situation that is likely to be, at least, unsettling for you. If your sensitivity to feeling rejected becomes extreme you might get **suspicious** of people whom you might have **brief paranoid thoughts** about. Your relationships might have a 'roller-coaster' quality to them—up or down rather than even and steady.

If you have BPD, it is likely that you did not have enough of the right opportunities to develop and learn the skills to deal with life problems and of ways of feeling good about yourself and the world. You might not have had the experiences of learning that difficult times can pass and that you can cope with being distressed. If this is the case, you will have been left with very high levels of distress without skills of how to deal with this distress other than engaging in **impulsive behaviours** that might make you feel better briefly but have long-term negative consequences. Examples of such impulsive behaviours might include verbal or physical attacks, **self-harm, alcohol, and other substance use, sex you later regretted, disordered eating, and excessive spending**. Another way that you might have developed of dealing with painful feelings is to **numb out**, including what professionals call **dissociation**. This numbing out might be contributing to your **lack of sense of your identity** and also your feelings of **emptiness**. Numbing out also means that you don't have the opportunities to practise and get skilful in dealing with emotions, resulting in **unstable emotions**.

Your recovery will include setting up structures so that you can have enough positive experiences to regulate your emotions, build a sense of who you are, your value and worth, and to learn skills of living that will enable you to enjoy the good times and to ride out the bad times as best you can without having to engage in impulsive behaviours that make things worse. Recovery will mean your being more skilled at managing your intense emotions, with less need to numb out, and your mood will consequently be more stable. Your behaviour will also be skilful whatever your mood. You will be aware of anger earlier on and use the information that anger brings to look after yourself. As you feel better about yourself, you will be less sensitive to feeling rejected and abandoned, better able to manage being alone without feeling empty, and better able to manage your life, your emotions, and your relationships relying on your own developing skills.

Like being romantically dumped non-stop!

Most people will have some of the features of BPD at some times in their lives without having BPD. A good example is how someone feels, thinks, and behaves after being romantically dumped. Having BPD is a bit like being romantically dumped except that you are likely to feel that way over many years—that is, the features are enduring and long-standing (the term 'like being romantically dumped' is used with the permission of Ruth E.S. Allen).

Sensitivity

Linehan (1993a) who developed a form of treatment known as dialectical behaviour therapy* (DBT) describes people with BPD often having:

- High sensitivity (quick emotional response to major and minor situations)

- High reactivity (emotional response is large)

- Slow return to baseline (emotional distress persists for a long time).

A number of people with BPD and clinicians have described the emotional sensitivity of people with BPD to be like that of the physical sensitivity of people with severe extensive burns. One of us (Roy) worked for a few months many years ago in a hospital burns unit. The physical pain of the patients was enormous, as you no doubt can imagine. The burns left people with understandable skin sensitivity where even slight changes such as the movement of sheets caused pain of a level that words could not communicate.

If you have BPD, there is a reasonable chance that you are a highly sensitive person. Sensitivity has relative strengths and weaknesses. Sensitivity might be part of your painful reactivity to emotional situations. On the other hand, in your recovery you will be using the strengths of your sensitivity to find out all you can about yourself and the world around you, so that you can find effective solutions to your problems.

All or nothing thinking

Beck *et al.* (1990) describes people with BPD often having three core ways of thinking (schema*):

- The world is dangerous and malevolent (wishing evil)

- I am powerless and vulnerable

- I am inherently unacceptable.

and describe how these core beliefs interface:

> Some persons who view the world as a dangerous, malevolent place believe that they can rely on their own strengths and abilities in dealing with the threats it presents. However, borderline individuals' belief that they are weak and powerless blocks this solution. Other individuals who believe that they are not capable of dealing effectively with the demands of daily life resolve their dilemma by becoming dependent on someone who they see as capable of taking care of them (and develop a dependent pattern). However, borderlines' belief that they are inherently unacceptable blocks this solution, since this belief leads them to conclude that dependence entails a serious risk of rejection, abandonment, or attack if this inherent unacceptability is discovered. Borderline individuals face quite a dilemma: convinced that they are relatively helpless in a hostile world but without a source of security, they are forced to vacillate between autonomy and dependence without being able to rely on either.
>
> Reprinted with the permission of Guilford Press

All or nothing (black and white) thinking refers to a tendency to see things in absolutes and is common in people with BPD. Examples that might apply to all of us include:

- loving someone one moment and hating them the next

- forgetting that people have both positive and negative features

- forgetting that people have both strengths and weaknesses

- forgetting that you have both strengths and weaknesses.

If you have ever felt that life is like a roller-coaster ride, this is one of the primary reasons. The world, people, and yourself rarely exist in absolute terms. Seeing the world, people, and yourself in all your and their full complexity without losing your sense of yourself will be part of your recovery.

Idealization and devaluation

This is discussed under 'Criterion 2' and 'all or nothing thinking'.

Strong sense of justice: aiming for justice at the expense of being effective

People with BPD are often sensitized to injustice because of the injustices of their past experiences. This can be associated with a determination for justice to prevail in all circumstances. This may apply to you. We believe our sense of justice needs to be valued, alongside valuing ourselves. Both justice and looking after ourselves are important. There are significant disadvantages in idealistically 'going down in a blaze of bullets' for a cause that does not justify the risks we are taking. It is important that you live to 'fight another day' and that 'winning the battle' is less important than winning the struggle to recovery.

Harsh on self (and others)

Perhaps related to seeing the world in absolute all or nothing ways is the anger you might feel for yourself and others when your expectations are not met. We have not met any single group of people who are consistently harder on themselves than people with BPD. This is a very sad irony. Many people with BPD have had very difficult pasts and are in need of a high level of self-acceptance. If the world were a fair place and justice prevailed, then people with BPD would, because of their difficult pasts, have a view of themselves that was compassionate, caring, and accepting. Unfortunately often quite the opposite occurs as we internalize the invalidating messages about ourselves that we have been given. This then results in a harsh view of ourselves and sometimes others. Recovery will include exploring how you can become caring and compassionate to yourself and to the important people in your life who you believe warrant caring and compassion.

Fluctuating competence

Some people with BPD can have times of high levels of competence only to decompensate rapidly following an event into a low level of competence. Some are competent in certain situations but unable to sustain this competence in other situations. This can be very difficult for yourself and others, and once again can be part of the roller-coaster ride of extreme ups and downs. Family and friends close to you may also be perplexed by this rapid change from competence to incompetence. It can also be disconcerting for strangers who are stunned by your sudden deterioration in competence. Recovery will include learning how to ride out distressing times while maintaining your competencies and also to strengthen and generalize your competencies so that you apply your competencies whatever your mood and across a wide range of situations. In short, recovery will aim for you being a consistent all-rounder.

Comment from Wendy

For a part of my recovery I was able to be incredibly functional in a work situation, but struggled immensely at the end of each working day. It was almost like I used all my resources up while at work and had none left when I was outside work. This was really hard to understand for me and others. Because I worked in the health field many of the professionals working with me could not understand how they saw a competent and capable person at work who was desperate and needing support outside of work. I often felt that they thought I was deliberately not coping at certain times of day. The fact was, that for me over that period with the clear expectations and goals in my working day, I well understood what was required of me, and how to 'be' or behave, and knew I was capable in that situation. I had none of those structures or reinforcements in my personal life, and could not manage that part of my life.

Active passivity

The term 'Active passivity' used by Linehan (1993a), refers to a situation where we actively work hard on being passive.

An example might include telling a person about a problem that we have and actively encouraging them to fix our problem or passively waiting for them to fix it. It makes sense that if we have not built a history of success doing things we will try get others to do things for us. This style can be effective at times in getting people to do things for us; however, if this is our dominant style it has the major downside of making sure that we will not be learning skills required for life.

Because of a lack of successes in the past we might be demoralized about our capacity ever to be successful at doing things. This will result in feelings of helplessness and resultant passivity. The desire to avoid what is perceived as yet another inevitable failure can understandably result in us being very active in ensuring we are passive. If we are passive and don't try something we might think that we can't fail at the task. To succeed at our recovery we obviously have to try and succeed at our recovery.

There are clear dangers if we are actively passive in our approach to our recovery and our therapy. Therapy at its best is a journey where both therapist and person-in-recovery are collaborating and both working actively and hard on understanding the problems and exploring solutions. In DBT this state is described as 'willingness'. In Section 2, we will be exploring how you and your therapist actively work together on understanding yourself and your problems and working on a solution to your problems.

> **If there was one thing only that you could take from this book, we would want it to be that you be active in your recovery**

 ## Comment from Wendy

I know that people perceived me as being 'actively passive' and seemed to think this was deliberate. The fact was, I did not believe I had the power to change, and the only way I could see myself getting out of the situation I was in, was for the situation to be changed by someone else, or for someone to remove or protect me from the situation. A huge turning point came when I started to take a small but active part in changing things (with lots of support from others) and realized that I could take control and change some things.

Returning to make sense of the DSM-IV diagnostic criteria: criterion by criterion

We have listed each of the nine DSM-IV diagnostic criteria as they appear in the DSM-IV followed by our comments.

> *Criterion 1. Frantic efforts to avoid real or imagined abandonment*

If for whatever reason (biological predisposition, psychological trauma) we did not have regular experiences of being securely attached to important people who would be able to assist us in dealing with our intense distress, it is likely that we will bring this experience into our adult world believing that important people may not be there for us when we need them. We might fear being left alone and helpless to face what we believe is a tough harsh world. This fear of abandonment will understandably result in 'frantic efforts to avoid real and imagined abandonment'. This may range from being as helpless as you can to expressing drastic thoughts of what will happen if they leave you that might encourage others to be there for you as you want them to be. This may prevent abandonment especially in the short term, but may also be destructive to the very relationship that you are trying to protect and actually drive the person away. Sometimes you may yourself end the relationship as a way of getting in first, thereby avoiding the imagined inevitable abandonment yourself.

 Comment from Wendy

I often caused myself a lot of distress by ending friendships or relationships if someone seemed angry or unhappy with me, because I believed they were going to walk out of my life, even if they were only a little angry with me. It was really important to me, that I took control and walked away first. I lost a lot of relationships like this. A major point for me was taking some small risks and hanging around when I thought someone was not happy with me, and discovering that most of the time their apparent crossness was either non-existent or unrelated to me. If it was related to me, it was often a simple misunderstanding that could be sorted with a quick conversation. The relationships with my friends and family that have negotiated what I now know are the ups and downs of normal relationships are one of the delights of my recovery.

Criterion 2. A pattern of unstable and intense interpersonal relationships characterized by alternating between extremes of idealization and devaluation

Do you put others on an elevated platform, seeing them as perfect—possibly perfect saviours and everything that you wished for—and later find yourself full of contempt for the person and hating them?

Young children often relate to important people in an all or nothing manner, seeing them one moment as perfect and after a real or imagined slight raging against them and hating them the next moment. Intense emotional experiencing can exacerbate this tendency, resulting in intense and unstable relationships as we have not yet learned to skilfully build in effective ways of celebrating and living with our emotional intensity. Without the right circumstances we are unlikely to develop the ability to see people as having both desirable and less desirable attributes. Given the right circumstances we can develop capacity to manage strong emotions and synthesize all or nothing idealization and devaluation and see people consistently as whole real life people who by nature have both strengths and weaknesses. These therapy tasks will be part of your recovery.

Comment from Wendy

I was an expert at putting people on a pedestal. I would meet somebody, and they were the answer to my dreams. Then they would turn out to be only human after all, and my image of the person was dashed—they were the most dreadful person in the world, and how could I have been such a bad judge of character. Many friendships were destroyed in this way, and one of the more satisfying parts of my recovery is being able to think to myself 'oh—Jane is having a bad day today', or 'Jill is awesome AND it annoys me when she . . . but hey our friendship is bigger than that'.

Criterion 3. Identity disturbance: markedly and persistently unstable self-image or sense of self

Are you often asking yourself questions like 'Who am I, what do I want from life, and what do I want to do with my life?' Do you search continuously for answers to these questions only to find that when you think you are getting to know what you want from life, you lose interest? This may be an outcome of unharnessed emotional intensity or it might be an understandable searching for what makes sense to us in a world that has not to date made that much sense. If our previous experience of emotions has been very painful we might have coped by shutting out as much feeling and as many emotions as we can. This may work for us to some degree, but may have the effect of leaving us feeling empty and uncertain about what we want from life.

 Comment from Wendy

For most of my life I had no idea who I was. I would suck up the identities of those around me. I would meet someone, and as mentioned above would think they were the perfect example of the human species. I would hang out with them, and do the things they did. At various points I was an active left-of-centre political party member, right-of-centre political party member, had short hair, long hair, liked country music, then rock, loved being a nurse, hated being a nurse, and on it went. I now have a strong sense of the values and things that are important to me—I wear the clothes I do, and my hair the way I do because that is who I am—if others don't like it—too bad!

> *Criterion 4. Impulsivity in at least two areas that are potentially self-damaging (e.g. spending, sex, substance abuse, reckless driving, binge eating). Note: do not include suicidal or self-mutilating behaviour covered in Criterion 5*

Impulsive behaviours arise when we are so distressed that we will do virtually anything to feel even a little bit better even if this only lasts a short while and even if it has serious long-term consequences. It is much like and includes being addicted to substances such as alcohol or heroin that briefly help us feel better in the short term but have serious negative consequences. If our lives are full of pain and we have yet to learn effective ways of dealing with our distress, then impulsive behaviours are understandable and very likely. Impulsive behaviours may include gambling, binge eating, driving recklessly, sex that is regretted, excessive spending, alcohol use, and other substance use.

Comment from Wendy

For many years, spending was something that gave me instant gratification. If I was feeling distressed, I would go shopping—frequently buying things I never used, and often not being able to pay essential bills. I would have some sense in the back of my mind that I might regret this later, but the need to feel better instantly was all encompassing. I still love spending, but now love not putting myself in debt for things that are not important and love being able to save and wait for things I really want.

> *Criterion 5. Recurrent suicidal behaviour, gestures or threats, or self mutilating behaviour*

This is mostly self-explanatory. Self-mutilating behaviour refers to harm deliberately inflicted upon the body usually as a means of relieving emotional distress, and can take many forms.

> *Criterion 6. Affective instability due to a marked reactivity of mood (e.g. intense episodic dysphoria, irritability or anxiety usually lasting a few hours and only rarely more than a few days)*

Do your emotions shift rapidly and unpredictably in response to internal or external cues or sometimes for reasons that you have yet to identify? This may seem like an intense roller-coaster ride with its rapid ups and downs but generally without the pleasure that people who enjoy roller-coaster rides experience. Also people who go on roller-coaster rides are in charge of and choosing to have the experience. Many people with BPD do not yet feel in control of their emotions but rather that emotions are controlling them. These experiences could be caused by your as yet unharnessed biological emotional intensity (brain chemistry that makes you sensitive and highly reactive to internal and external cues/triggers), idealization, devaluation (all or nothing) previously described, or by the numerous internal or external cues that can lead to you feeling intensely, or by any combination of these.

Criterion 7. Chronic feelings of emptiness

Emptiness may result for a number of different reasons. Understandably, if our lives have involved numerous disappointments we may become fearful of trying things and fearful of engaging in life; we may avoid a lot of things to try to decrease our distress. Unfortunately this is likely to leave us with not enough going on in our life that is meaningful. Shutting out emotions will leave us without the ability to know what is meaningful and satisfying—empty. Attempts to fill this emptiness while either avoiding engaging in life or blocking the experience of emotions may be to no avail. This is like trying to fill a bucket with water when the bucket has holes in the base. Emptiness is also likely to result from difficulties establishing and maintaining satisfying intimate relationships that would otherwise fill/fulfil us. Recovery will involve developing skills and relationships that will mend the hole in the bucket.

Comment from Wendy

It was not until I read the diagnostic criteria for BPD that I was able to put words to the big hole inside me. I felt that I was hollow and worthless, and that my existence had no meaning or substance. Later, I needed to be constantly active to fill the black hole in me. To this day, I do not like to spend long periods of time unoccupied—a sense of purpose is very important to me.

Criterion 8. Inappropriate intense anger or difficulty controlling anger (e.g. frequent displays of temper, constant anger, recurrent physical fights)

Are you easily cued into rages like some people experience with 'road rage'? Anger may be experienced by all of us in response to our experience of frustrated needs and experience of disappointment, and can be a very powerful experience that may be overwhelming. Having a biological brain that experiences emotions intensely can prime us to intense anger. Also, if our world view is that important people should be perfect and able to meet our every need, then it will be inevitable that we will be enraged when others fall from this unsustainable lofty pedestal that we have placed them on. Being angry in itself is usually not a problem; it is the behaviour resulting from the angry feelings that determines whether we are acting in our best interests or against our best interests. For example, punching somebody that results in us going to jail is likely to be against our interests and the person we punched. Just because somebody does not like us being angry or because they cannot understand the intensity of our anger does not make the anger 'inappropriate'. The term 'inappropriate' refers to behaviours consequent to angry feelings that lead to problems for ourselves and perhaps others. Anger is just one of a number of emotions that can have important functions (such as protecting us from real danger). Recovery will involve learning skills to harness this energy in an effective and productive way.

Criterion 9. Transient, stress related paranoid ideation or severe dissociative symptoms

---

If we have had past experiences of feeling misunderstood by people or, worse, that people have been dangerous (e.g. physical/sexual assault), it will be likely that we will be supersensitive to and highly watchful for danger. This will serve us really well in telling the difference between safe and unsafe people but may let us down when we over-react to events, perceiving danger when none exists—that can be called paranoid thinking. We may have a wariness and suspicion of people which, while understandable in terms of our past experiences, might cause problems for ourselves. This may manifest by avoiding contact with people or raging against people whom we later recognize as having done us no wrong. In this way we might avoid building bridges in relationships or alternatively leave behind us a series of destroyed bridges and relationships that are difficult to repair.

You may be someone who 'numbs out' intentionally or unintentionally as a way of not feeling. Dissociation is a way of not feeling and may take the form of 'feeling numb', 'switching out' to more extreme forms where no memory occurs for an event or events.

5

Other problems or diagnoses found in association with borderline personality disorder

> **➲ Key points**
>
> ◆ If you have BPD, the chances are you will also have or have had about three to four other diagnoses.
>
> ◆ It is only a minority of people with BPD who have 'pure' BPD with no other diagnoses.
>
> ◆ This information guides treatment.

We understand BPD best as a collection of features that professionals categorize into a 'diagnosis'. If you have BPD and have had an ongoing and constant difficult time throughout your life it will not be the least bit surprising if you get depressed or anxious or use a variety of means such as self-harm, substance abuse, and binge eating to deal with your distress. When a professional categorizes these symptoms and behaviours they may come up with a number of diagnoses. If you have BPD, the chances are you will also have or have had about three to four other diagnoses. It is only a minority of people with BPD who have 'pure' BPD with no other diagnoses. We list (Table 5.1) some of the more common mental health diagnoses associated with BPD with brief descriptions and a percentage figure with which this diagnosis has been shown in different studies to occur in people with BPD.

Table 5.1 Some of the more common mental health diagnoses associated with BPD

Depressive disorder* (35–85%): usually refers to being depressed for a distinct time period.
Dysthymic disorder* (25–65%): refers to being depressed for long periods (more than 2 years) at a lower level usually than with a depressive disorder.
Bipolar disorder/bipolar affective disorder* (uncertain, perhaps 1–15%): condition typically characterized by episodes of depression and mania (excessively elevated or irritable mood, racy thoughts, and other features often requiring hospitalization). Bipolar II disorder* refers to a condition with episodes of depression and hypomania (features like those of mania that are of shorter duration or do not require hospitalization).
Generalized anxiety disorder* (10%): anxious in many areas of life.
Panic disorder* (30–50%): time-limited (usually less than 30 min) overwhelming episodes of anxiety.
Agoraphobia* (10–35%): anxiety—usually about being in unfamiliar situations.
Social phobia* (25–50%): anxiety about social situations usually with significant avoidance of social situations.
Post-traumatic stress disorder* (35–55%): anxiety clearly linked with a psychological trauma, often with invasive memories of the trauma and an excessively high level of general watchfulness and alertness.
Obsessive-compulsive disorder* (15–25%): anxiety due to intrusive irrational thoughts that the person recognizes as their own followed by a 'compulsion' activity that serves to decrease the anxiety although the activity is recognized as irrational. For example, irrational fears of germs resulting in hand washing.
Alcohol and other substance dependence or abuse* (20–65%): physical dependence or problems related to alcohol or other substance use.
Bulimia* (25–40%): binge eating associated with unhealthy behaviours preventing weight gain such as fasting, vomiting, purgative/laxative usage, and excess exercise.
Binge eating disorder*: binge eating without unhealthy behaviours preventing weight gain such as fasting, vomiting, purgative/laxative usage, and excess exercise. (see 'Bulimia' above for comparison).
Eating disorder (any eating disorder—30–50%)

Krawitz and Watson (2003); Zanarini *et al.* (2004a).

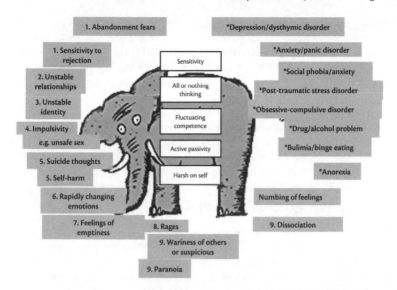

Figure 5.1. Understanding BPD: BPD DSM-IV criteria reworded[1–9] and other problems or diagnoses* associated with BPD. Adapted from and printed with the permission of Kiera Van Gelder, President, Middle Path, consumer organization dedicated to the advocacy, support, and education of those affected by BPD.

Figure 5.1 is an adaptation from a colleague, Kiera van Gelder who has used the parable of the elephant to illustrate various features of BPD. In the parable, various blind people touching an elephant, were asked to describe what an elephant was and described the elephant completely differently. One person holding a tusk described the elephant as a plough another holding a foot as a pillar and another holding the tail as a brush. It is the same with BPD. Up close we may see some parts in great detail but not others and need to step back to be able to see all of what the BPD condition may involve. On the left-hand side are the DSM-IV features of BPD reworded into regular non-professional language, on the right-hand side, some of the commonly associated problems and diagnoses and in the centre some of the ways of understanding BPD described earlier.

Suicide

Thoughts of suicide are very common in people with BPD. Often these thoughts are around for quite a long time, with periods of greater intensity. The suicide rate is significant, with older studies suggesting a suicide rate of 10%. More recent studies are suggestive of a substantially lower figure. As newer, more effective treatments are being provided, it would make sense that the suicide rate would lessen. This is certainly our experience.

Overlap with depression

There is a considerable relationship between BPD and depressive disorder*
and dysthymic disorder* that is vigorously debated but not yet resolved. At a
treatment level it will not be surprising if you are depressed in one way or
another at least for some of the time. While antidepressant medication is
appropriate for treatment for a depressive disorder that you may have, it
is very important that you are also engaged in therapy as the response to anti-
depressants of people who are depressed who have BPD is thought by most
experts, but not all, to be less than that which occurs with people with a
depressive disorder who do not have a BPD diagnosis.

Overlap with bipolar disorder*

There is overlap between the symptoms of BPD and bipolar affective disorder*
(previously known as manic depressive disorder). When the differential diagnosis (the list of possible diagnoses) includes BPD and bipolar affective disorder,
accurate diagnosis where possible will greatly improve outcome. Accurate diagnosis of bipolar disorder will usually mean that medication treatment will have a
major role in treatment planning. Accurate diagnosis of BPD on the other hand
will lead to a somewhat different treatment plan where therapy is the dominant
treatment. The presenting symptoms of BPD can be remarkably similar to those
of a brittle, rapidly fluctuating form of bipolar disorder. Compared with people
with bipolar disorder, people with BPD have emotional shifts that tend to be of
shorter duration, of more rapid onset and termination, and more immediately
linked to an identifiable environmental stressor with a strong interpersonal context. Sometimes people can have both BPD and bipolar disorder.

 Comment from Wendy

I was very disappointed and had to work hard at emotionally accepting it,
when after a few years of not needing mental health treatment, I again
required treatment for a newly developed bipolar disorder*. I am aware
that there can be great difficulty distinguishing BPD and bipolar disorder*
presentations for some people. However, for me the two disorders were
classically different in presentation as outlined in the paragraph above and
in Table 5.1 of this chapter. Increasing scientific awareness of the higher
than expected occurrence of bipolar disorder* in people with BPD has left
me wondering whether for me there may have been common biological
(and perhaps psychological) causal factors.

Interface with psychosis

The interface between psychotic experiences and BPD has generated considerable debate; however, the area remains unresolved. The presence of psychotic* symptoms, while inviting consideration of a diagnosis of schizophrenia* or bipolar disorder*, is not sufficient for the diagnosis. 'Psychotic' symptoms broadly refer to having delusions (fixed false beliefs not in keeping with our cultural context) and/or hallucinations (voice/s of somebody speaking with no objective evidence of that person being around). Transient paranoid thinking is one of the DSM-IV diagnostic criteria for BPD. The presence of hallucinosis (a type of hallucination where the person knows that the voice being heard originates from themselves and not externally) and brief psychotic episodes are not unusual in people meeting diagnostic criteria for BPD without the person meeting any of the other diagnostic criteria for schizophrenia.

Incorrect diagnosis

There are dangers in making an incorrect diagnosis. An incorrect diagnosis of BPD may deprive you of medication treatment that is rapidly effective and relatively easy to introduce, for example, for bipolar disorder or schizophrenia. On the other hand an incorrect diagnosis of bipolar disorder encourages an excessive focus on medication treatments compared with psychological treatments. A positive diagnosis of BPD is ideally made without it being a diagnosis of exclusion (when all other diagnoses have been tried and eliminated), or a failure to respond to medications.

Overlap with other personality disorders

BPD is one of 11 personality disorder categories defined in DSM-IV. If we meet diagnostic criteria for BPD there is a fair chance we will meet diagnostic criteria for another personality disorder. This is not meant to alarm you but highlights the fact that the personality disorder categories, not surprisingly, often overlap significantly.

The more commonly associated personality disorders are defined in Table 5.2 with the percentage figures referring to the likelihood of having that particular personality disorder if we have BPD. The two most common associated personality disorders are probably avoidant and dependent followed by paranoid and antisocial personality disorder.

Table 5.2 The more commonly associated personality disorders

Avoidant personality disorder (35–45%): personality style of excessive avoiding of stressful life situations that causes problems (e.g. avoiding anxiety-provoking social situations, leading to loneliness).

Dependent personality disorder (40–50%): personality style of excessive relying on others that leads to difficulties (e.g. leaning on others for decision-making maintains low self-belief and leaves dependent person vulnerable when the other person is not around).

Paranoid personality disorder (20–30%): excessive wariness and suspicion of others that causes problems.

Antisocial personality disorder (15–25%): engaging in behaviours that impact on people in ways that society finds unacceptable (repeated violation of the rights of others).

From Zanarini *et al.,* (1998, 2004b)

It is not in the least surprising that paranoid, avoidant, and dependent personality disorder are associated with BPD as these are perfectly understandable responses to difficult pasts. If we have not been understood or have been abused by others it is completely understandable and not in the least surprising that we will be wary of people. If we have been unsuccessful in past activities, avoiding situations is an understandable way of coping with high anxiety, albeit problematic. If we have low self-confidence it makes sense, albeit problematic, that we will look to others for solutions to life's problems. Of course, saying that it is understandable, is not passive resigned acceptance of the situation, but on the contrary, could be the basis for change, should we wish to change.

6

What causes borderline personality disorder?

> **⊃ Key points**
>
> ◆ Most international experts are in agreement that biological and psychological factors can contribute to the development of the condition and that there is often interplay between these biological and psychological factors.
>
> ◆ Socio-cultural factors may interact with biological and psychological protective and risk factors, increasing or decreasing the likelihood of BPD developing.
>
> ◆ The pathway to developing the disorder will be unique for you, with different predisposing or protecting factors from biological, psychological, and socio-cultural sources.
>
> ◆ Whatever the causes in your unique situation, treatment effectiveness requires both you and your treating clinician/s being very active in your treatment.

The chances are that you are interested in understanding causes of BPD. Reaching an understanding of the unique causes for you can be experienced as validating and often enables people (people with BPD and their families) to move on to present and future solutions and recovery. It is important to note, however, that there is no single cause for BPD and for most it will be an interplay of the factors discussed here.

Biological factors

Research has shown that if you have BPD you are statistically more likely to have brain functioning different from people without the condition. The most notable of these differences is what is referred to as a 'sluggish serotonin system'. What this means is that if you were given a chemical substance under laboratory conditions that usually kick starts the serotonin system into action, the response of your serotonin system, if you have BPD would more probably be 'sluggish' than if you did not have BPD. Sluggish serotonin systems are statistically associated with lowered mood, depression, irritability, anger, and impulsivity.

There is some research showing people with BPD to be more likely to have smaller volumes of two parts of the brain associated with managing stress (amygdala and hippocampus) and to have a different brain response to stress.

It is not known at this stage whether these physiological and anatomical brain differences are a predisposition to developing BPD, a response to life experiences, or some combination of these two factors.

DBT hypothesizes that people with BPD may be born with a biological predisposition of being people who experience emotion more intensely (emotionally sensitive) than the rest of the population. This is neither good nor bad and has advantages and disadvantages. If parents themselves do not experience emotions as intensely, it will understandably be difficult for them to know what the experience of emotional intensity is like and will not have had the personal experience of successfully making the most out of this temperament. It would be hard for any parent in these circumstances to model how to deal with intense emotions or how to teach their child to work with their intense emotions. So, the sad situation here is that even the most caring of parents may be unable to teach their child how to celebrate, work with, and manage their intense emotions. If this happens, the child may feel misunderstood, which will then impact on the parents who may feel ineffective at parenting and a cycle of misunderstanding may become embedded. We have heard parents describe feeling powerless at not knowing how to assist their sensitive child in their childhood and how this led to great difficulties for all parties. We have seen parents and their adult children in tears of joy (and sadness of lost years) on hearing and discussing this explanation of cause, shifting to a position of neither parents nor adult child being to blame, moving beyond blame to solutions. These have been some of the most moving and rewarding events that we have witnessed as parent and adult child come to understand that nobody was to blame and that all parties were doing the best they knew how. This can set the stage for all parties to move on to solutions in the present and future.

It is increasingly recognized that there is a substantial genetic contribtion to personality. This may include factors such as high emotional intensity, high emotional sensitivity, high emotional reactivity and higher levels of impulsivity, irritability, and novelty-seeking. It is thought that abour 50% of personality is inherited. One large study (Torgerson *et al.*, 2000) of identical and non-identical twins of people with BPD showed that the identical twins had a 35% chance of having BPD, whereas the non-identical twins had only a 7% chance of having BPD. This strongly suggests that genetics has a significant contribution. (A much smaller earlier twin study did not demonstrate a likelihood of BPD being inherited, possibly due to the small study size.)

Another study of people diagnosed with a depressive disorder showed that 8% of people without a particular gene and without a history of childhood sexual abuse had a history of self-harm. This rose to 30–36% either where the gene was present or where there was a history of childhood sexual abuse and to 60% where both the gene was present and there was a history of childhood sexual abuse (Joyce *et al.*, 2006). The conclusions of this study are that both biological and psychological factors contribute to self-harm, which is most frequent when both biological and psychological factors exist.

Psychological factors

Being brought up in an environment that was abusive or neglectful will obviously have a profound impact on our psychological development decreasing our chances of entering adulthood with psychological skills, good self-esteem, and confidence. People with BPD report a high incidence of past physical and sexual abuse, childhood neglect, and childhood emotional deprivation. You may well have a history of sexual abuse. Sexual abuse is clearly a risk factor for developing the condition, with about 70% of people with BPD reporting a history of sexual abuse. However, you may not have a history of sexual abuse. Thirty per cent of people with BPD do not report a history of sexual abuse. Also, the majority of people who are sexually abused do not go on to develop BPD.

Nature and nurture: interplay of biological and psychological factors

Most international experts are in agreement that biological and psychological factors can contribute to the development of the condition and that there is often interplay between these biological and psychological factors. However, there is dispute regarding the relative contributions of these two factors. A large amount of information now exists that the debate of nature versus nurture is now outdated and has been replaced with 'nature and nurture, nature via nurture, or nurture via nature'.

Is BPD an illness?

You may be wondering whether BPD is an illness. We do not have a yes or no answer to this question and hope the above discussion provides you with background information related to this question. At the end of the day, what is most important is that you receive effective treatment and recover. To this end, you will recall that psychological therapy is the dominant recommended treatment for BPD, with biological treatments (medication) having an assisting role. If we have an illness such as pneumonia, then it is appropriate that we are relatively passive waiting for treating clinicians to fix us (even here we can contribute to our recovery by, for example, active involvement in self-help physiotherapy instructions). It is absolutely critical that you do not get into a passive position if you have BPD. Treatment effectiveness requires both you and your treating clinician/s being very active in your treatment whatever the causal factors in your unique situation are.

Socio-cultural factors

Many people believe that there are socio-cultural factors that protect or predispose to developing BPD. It has been suggested that risk factors include changed and changing social roles and expectations, loss of the extended family, societal breakdown, and substance use cultures. The suggested protective factors include a connected intact society, clear role expectations, extended family networks, and cultures that place high value on interpersonal attachment and connection.

Unique set of multiple interacting factors

The pathway to developing the disorder will be unique for you, with different predisposing or protecting factors from biological, psychological, and socio-cultural sources.

For example, some people will have had a high genetic predisposition and required only a small environmental contribution to push past the threshold (barrier) for having BPD. On the other hand, another person may have had few genetic predisposing factors but had such devastating trauma (such as repeated ongoing childhood sexual abuse from an early age) that this was sufficient to push through the threshold. If you were sexually abused this will obviously be a likely predisposing factor. If the sexual abuse occurred as a child, how people that you shared this with responded could have been predisposing or protective. A validating response where people were believing, very supportive, and ensured that the abuse never happened again would have been somewhat protective compared with an invalidating response where you were not believed, not supported, and not protected from further abuse.

Socio-cultural factors may interface with biological and psychological protective and risk factors, increasing or decreasing the likelihood of BPD developing. For example, having a supportive caring validating extended family member such as a grandparent might decrease the likelihood for developing BPD.

You may have no history of childhood abuse or neglect and you and your parents are stuck, unable to move beyond blame on to solutions, as you grapple with finding a convincing way of understanding causal factors. A way through this stalemate may be that you might have been born sensitive (biological) and that your parents did the best that they could. The quality of the parenting you received might well have been sufficient for other children born less sensitive (perhaps including brothers and sisters) but was unfortunately insufficient for you, born sensitive. This understanding might assist moving beyond blame towards solutions. These solutions include recognizing and validating an ongoing biological vulnerability and mutually validating interactions that result in upward spiralling transactions between you and those close to you. There is also a growing body of evidence in the field of mental health suggesting that improved psychological well-being can also result in an upward spiral of improved brain function. This in turn can influence interpersonal transactions, and so on.

A suggested pathway that might apply to you could have a starting point of being born with predisposing physiology such as high emotional experiencing and/or childhood emotional trauma. As a consequence of either or both of these factors, relationships were affected and physiology and possibly brain 'hard wiring' altered, decreasing learning capacity and increasing impulsivity, emotional instability, and sensitivity to stress. This, in turn, impacted on relationships, which in turn affected brain function, and so on. High sensitivity and reactivity to emotional events, unstable emotions, identity problems, relationship problems, poor self-image, and counter-productive self-talk resulted and in time the behaviours and internal experiences of someone meeting diagnostic criteria for BPD developed.

Why are more females diagnosed with BPD?

There are a number of possible theories as to why females outweigh males:

♦ The incidence of sexual abuse is reported to be higher among females.

♦ Girls and women living in a marginalized, invalidating environment.

- The diagnosis being gender biased (the diagnosis is based on emotional expressivity, which is higher among females).

- Females may be taught more than males to value relationships, leaving females more vulnerable to a condition defined by relationship difficulties.

- Males with psychological problems seek out professional help less frequently.

- Males with the same behaviours are more likely to receive a diagnosis of antisocial personality disorder.

- Males with the same factors causing the difficulties may be more likely to be found in substance use services and to externalize their anger and end up in the justice system. There are strong suggestions that a significant percentage of perpetrators of family violence (who are more frequently male) would meet diagnostic criteria for BPD, if assessed.

 Comment from Wendy

In making the following comment, I am working from what I consider two entirely reasonable assumptions.

- We are not responsible for our genes

- As children we are not primarily responsible for the quality of the relationships that we had with adults during our childhood

Assuming these to be accurate, we can then say:

- How we entered adulthood was a result of our genes, biological temperament, and our experience of childhood

- It is logical to assume that how we entered adulthood is largely not our fault

However, if we entered adulthood with difficulties, we need to take control by learning new ways of being and new skills to make for ourselves the life we want. Linehan, the developer of DBT, writes that people '… may not have caused all of their own problems, but they have to solve them anyway' (Linehan, 1993a, p. 107).

7

Understanding self-harm

 Key points

- For the purposes of our discussion, we are defining self-harm as deliberate behaviours intended to do physical harm to the body without intent to die, that serve a short-term function but have negative long-term consequences.

- We have deliberately not outlined the specific behaviours of self-harm as we wish to focus attention rather on alternative solutions to the feelings that precipitate self-harm behaviour.

- Common short-term functions of self-harm can be divided into two broad groups:
  - dealing with internal distress directly
  - dealing with internal distress indirectly by effects on external environment.

Therapy tasks include:

- Finding ways of avoiding self-harm including alternative behaviours

- Developing skills for dealing with cues that would previously have led to self-harm.

What is meant by the term self-harm?

For the purposes of our discussion we are defining self-harm as follows:

- Engaging in deliberate behaviours intended to do physical harm to the body without intending to die

- Behaviour serves a function in the short-term

- Behaviour has negative long-term consequences.

Common short-term functions of self-harm can be divided into two broad groups:

i) dealing with internal distress directly

ii) dealing with internal distress indirectly by effects on external environment.

Dealing with internal distress directly

- to feel better
- to change emotional pain into physical pain
- to make 'invisible' emotional pain visible
- to distract
- to deal with high anxiety
- to deal with high levels of anger
- to punish oneself
- to feel something
- to feel alive
- to not feel, feel numb or dissociate
- to prevent feeling numb or dissociated
- to feel grounded or whole
- to feel in control
- to care for oneself (e.g. look after wound caringly).

In these situations, self-harm is a private action. The purpose of the self-harm is achieved without anybody having to know about the self-harm.

Almost all of us deliberately engage in some behaviours that serve a short-term purpose but have negative long-term effects. Many of these behaviours are common in the general population and, perhaps for this reason, do not get labelled as self-harm. Examples of such behaviours include smoking, alcohol misuse, unhealthy eating, too much chocolate, overeating, undereating, too much exercise, too little exercise, and staying up too late at night.

Dealing with internal distress indirectly by effects on external environment

- ◆ to communicate to others
- ◆ to communicate intensity of distress to others
- ◆ to feel heard
- ◆ to attract caring responses from others
- ◆ to get access to mental health services
- ◆ to control others
- ◆ to punish others.

In these situations, self-harm is a public action. The purpose of the self-harm can only be achieved if others know about the self-harm.

Should I be concerned about my self-harm behaviours?

We assume that if you are engaging in self-harm behaviours, there will be a very understandable reason or reasons for this. In some way the self-harm behaviours are probably serving a purpose of helping you feel a little less distressed even if only for a very short time. So you might be thinking – well if it works for me then why stop? This is an excellent question. In addition to the obvious risks and damage to your physical health, self-harm behaviours can deprive us of opportunities for recovery and healing. One of the tasks in therapy is to find alternative behaviours that will serve the same and in time even better function as self-harm in decreasing emotional pain whilst at the same time also being good for you long-term. Another task is to identify cues, thoughts, behaviours and emotions that lead to self-harm, and then explore alternative solutions along the cascade of events that previously would have led to self-harm. This way you not only stop self-harming but very importantly learn effective ways of dealing with life situations and your thoughts and emotions.

We have deliberately not outlined the specific behaviours of self-harm as we wish to focus attention rather on alternative solutions to the feelings that precipitate self-harm behaviour.

Comment from Wendy

Sometimes people feel a lot of shame or guilt when they self-harm. It is important that you do not make things worse by giving yourself a hard time because you self-harm, but instead accept that this is where you are for now and work on alternative ways of dealing with the same cues or emotions.

8

Prognosis: do people with borderline personality disorder get better?

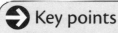 **Key points**

♦ In general, people get better!

Yes—an emphatic yes—people with BPD do generally get better!

What recovery means will be different for each person. For some it may be a decrease in distressing symptoms to the point where you are able to say that you feel that your life is worth living on more days than earlier. For others it may be feeling that your life is worth living on more days than not. For many people it is much more than this. Feeling connected to others and feeling that you have a valuable place in your community, whatever that might be for you, might be achicvable. The perfect life, with no issues or problems, is not a reality, but looking forward to each day, each year and your life ahead is.

If you have BPD, you will have been distressed for a number of years, and because change takes time it is easy to think that change is not possible. Change is definitely possible. Wendy is personal testament to this and we both have been witness to many people's recovery. We will now outline the scientific basis for the fact that recovery is achievable.

Zanarini *et al.* (2005) followed up people attending a private US mental health service known for its BPD treatment. At 6-year follow-up, 68% of those initially diagnosed with BPD no longer met diagnostic criteria for BPD and of those that had ever recovered (not meeting diagnostic criteria), only 6% had ever relapsed. The overwhelming majority (94%) of those that recovered stayed recovered (Zanarini *et al.*, 2005). This recent study by Zanarini *et al.* was extended to 10-year follow-up (Zanarini *et al.*, 2006) by which time about 85% of people initially diagnosed with BPD no longer met diagnostic criteria. These results are far more optimistic than views on prognosis a few decades ago.

Does time heal?

Earlier studies following people for a long period of time show that people do improve with the passage of time. Researchers believe that this was not just a direct result of treatment but also a feature of time specifically. This improving over time is thought to be related both to biological changes over time that result in decreased impulsivity and also to gradual learning of psychological skills over time.

 Comment from Wendy

When I was diagnosed with BPD, my first reaction was one of hopelessness—my prior knowledge was that there was no effective treatment—for a long time there was no research indicating otherwise. Fortunately I was lucky enough to have some wonderful clinicians who fully believed in my ability to get better—mostly they believed more than I did, and often it was only their belief in my ability to have a life that kept me going. The really exciting thing is that their belief in my ability to recover was not a false hope, and now there is research available to confirm this. It is likely that with modern treatments you will get better—the research says so!

9

Is treatment effective?

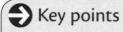 Key points

- Treatment can be effective!
- Expert agreement is that psychotherapy is the primary treatment for BPD with medication to assisty.

Of course if you are engaged in an effective treatment you are likely to recover more fully and faster than you would just with the passage of time. When science explores whether a treatment is effective, all the outcomes are pooled (joined) together. This means that science will report an analysis of the averages of all outcomes. So, when we write about an effective treatment, it means that if you are involved in this treatment there is a statistically similar chance of you achieving the same outcome. However, as in any group some people will have better and worse outcomes than others, which affect the averages reported.

Also, what works for one person will not necessarily work for another. So, do not give up if you have tried one treatment but not others. However, once you make a commitment to a particular treatment, we encourage you to stay with that treatment for a long enough period to assess whether that treatment will be effective for you. It is unlikely that it will be helpful to be engaged in a series of short treatments measured in terms of weeks.

Some of you may have had years of treatment and continue to be significantly distressed. Do not give up. Research has shown that change in many areas of human endeavour may take several attempts before being successful at another attempt. This is well recognized in the area of addictions including, for example, people addicted to nicotine, alcohol, or heroin who have successfully changed their behaviours and stopped smoking, using alcohol, or using heroin after previous unsuccessful efforts. If you have had unsuccessful previous treatment/s, do not give yourself a hard time but rather focus on what you can do this time around that will increase the likelihood of recovery and give it your best shot.

Expert agreement is that psychotherapy is the primary treatment for BPD, with medication assisting. The next paragraphs outline the scientific evidence that psychotherapy treatment can be effective, followed by an outline of the effectiveness of medication treatment.

Is psychotherapy treatment effective?

The first scientific research showing that psychotherapy treatment was effective was published in 1991. By mid-2007, there were 15 published studies of the highest scientific standard (randomized controlled trial* or controlled trial*). In addition there have been numerous other published studies of a lower level of scientific robustness (open uncontrolled trial*). Fifteen studies is a small number of studies but it is nevertheless conclusive that there is now a solid scientific evidence base that treatment of BPD can be effective. The numbers of studies published are increasing and we can look forward to ever growing evidence of psychotherapy treatment effectiveness. The uncontrolled trials* are of a lower scientific standard but are really important in demonstrating the practicality and feasibility of providing effective treatment outside of research settings in 'real world' situations, which is where you are most likely to be receiving treatment.

Nine of the 15 randomized controlled* or controlled trials* have used DBT* (see Chapter 11) as the treatment provided in three different research centres in North America and Europe. Five of the remaining trials have used four different variations of psychodynamic* or psychoanalytical* treatment (see Chapter 11) in four different centres in North America, the UK, and Australia, and there has been one randomized controlled trial demonstrating the effectiveness of schema-focused therapy. There has been one scientific trial (randomized controlled trial) of effective treatment using cognitive analytical therapy (see Chapter 11) for adolescents (most with BPD traits*, some with BPD) that is yet to be published due to the study being just completed. Preliminary data from this study demonstrates that high quality standard treatment (manual-based 'good clinical care') was also effective. Additional less scientific (uncontrolled) trials of DBT have shown its effectiveness in state-funded community programmes in different continents, one of which in New Hampshire, USA was awarded an American Psychiatric Association Gold Achievement Award for outstanding mental health programmes.

Obviously it makes sense to be involved in a treatment that has been shown to be effective. So if you can access any of the evidence-based effective treatments provided by clinicians who have an interest and experience in working with people with BPD, then do so. The finding that high quality standard treatment (manual-based 'good clinical care') carried out by clinicians interested and experienced in working with people with BPD can be effective means that this provides you with another viable treatment option to aim for which might be available to you when DBT, BPD relevant psychodynamic*/psychoanalytical* therapy, schema-focused therapy, or cognitive analytical therapy is not available.

Is medication treatment effective?

There is no single magical pill that will cure all people with BPD. Medications can be very effective for some people in treating some associated conditions such as depression and anxiety/panic attacks.

Specifically regarding the features of BPD, a range of medications have been shown to be effective in reducing some of the difficulties that people with BPD have by decreasing some of the following: impulsivity, irritability, anger, and emotional instability. In general, the medications do not result in a cure or full recovery from BPD features but can in many people take the edge off some of the more disabling symptoms. Some people have a more substantial response to medication treatment. The medications in common current use that have been shown statistically to be of some benefit in research studies are SSRIs (e.g. fluoxetine) and newer antipsychotic medication (e.g. olanzapine). Other newer medications with some evidence of effectiveness are the anticonvulsant topiramate, a newer antipsychotic, aripiprazole (one trial only), and the dietary supplement, omega 3 (one trial only). The scientific proof for other mood-stabilizing medication is lower (sodium valproate, carbamazepine). The strict conditions required for research studies (e.g. excluding people who are depressed) might account for some researchers commenting that clinical outcomes with the medications are not as positive as the outcomes achieved in research studies. There are no studies that we are aware of studying the effectiveness of medication taken occasionally at times of crisis only. In Section 2 we will explore how you might integrate this research knowledge as you consider the role of medication in your recovery.

Section 2

Recovery frameworks

In Section 2, we provide information to assist you to set up frameworks and structures for your effective treatment, recovery, and healing, whatever type of therapy you are engaged in. These frameworks include believing you can recover, getting yourself ready for change, selecting a therapist and taking charge of your recovery, making the most out of treatment that is available to you. If your therapist is learning about BPD, you may want to use this book collaboratively with your therapist.

10

Change

⊃ Key points

♦ Research on the science of psychological change shows that people who change tend to go through a reasonably predictable spiralling cycle.

♦ Hope—looking 'for a favourable outcome within the realm of possibilities' (Clarke, 2003).

♦ There are recognized ways of preparing for change, increasing the likelihood that change will take place as wanted.

♦ There are a number of different ways that you can acquire confidence that change is possible.

♦ There are key questions you can ask yourself about change.

Stages of change

Research on the science of psychological change shows that people tend to go through a reasonably predictable spiralling cycle as they consider and engage in positive change. This cycle is referred to as the Stages of change as outlined in Fig. 10.1.

As you can see in the figure, change often involves small steps, moving from a place of not even thinking about or wanting change (pre-contemplation) to ambivalently thinking about the advantages and disadvantages of change (contemplation), to preparation for taking action and then to taking action. The rest of the cycle of maintenance is in the form of an ongoing spiral to

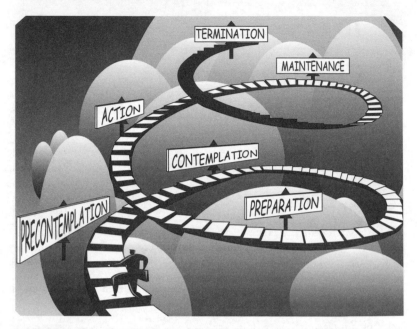

Figure 10.1. The spiral of change. Reproduced with permission from Harper Collins publishers. Copyright © by James O. Prochaska, John C. Norcross, and Carlo C. DiClemente.

emphasize that change requires ongoing work to maintain and that most of us will slip in some way at some point.

As slips are predictable we can work hard on trying to prevent slips and also get back on the change pathway when we do slip. Obviously we all aim not to slip and it is great if we do not slip. However, it is important that we have a compassionate way of looking at ourselves when we do slip and also be prepared for slips. It is important that a slip is seen as just that—a slip in an overall pathway of recovery—not a catastrophe. Two steps forward and one step back. We need to see a slip not as reason for giving up but rather as a signal to re-focus our attention on getting back on track as soon as we can and use the slip as a learning opportunity for our future recovery. Also, if we feel stuck despite our best efforts at change we will need to be compassionate with ourselves, accepting our stuckness while exploring how to become unstuck. A lot of work in the recovery from BPD is not only changing what we can but also accepting that sometimes things are not the way we would like. This can apply to slips or stuckness and strangely enough rather than preventing change may actually help us change due to the compassionate way of relating to ourselves, provided we do not excessively and/or permanently accept things that we can change.

Sometimes we will need to move from the action stage and return to the contemplation stage. The stages are not all or nothing, so we might find that we can benefit from work on pros and cons of change and on preparation for action and action at the same time.

Knowing the stage that we are in can assist the steps we can successfully take. If we are in the contemplation stage we need to explore the pros and cons of change. To advance towards change we will need to be open to or actively explore increasing our perceptions of the pros of change and the cons of not changing. You might achieve this by reading about BPD that is hopeful and encouraging of recovery, getting in touch with somebody who has recovered from BPD, or speaking to friends, family, and therapist about the pros and cons of change. If you have decided that you definitely want to change and believe that change is possible then you are in the preparation stage and need to develop a plan of action. Once you have a plan of action you need to move into the action stage and actually take action.

Example of pros and cons of change

Cons of not changing	Pros of not changing
Life sucks	Somebody will look after me
Relationships don't work	Cannot fail if I don't try
Cons of changing	**Pros of changing**
I have to put in so much effort	Living a satisfying life

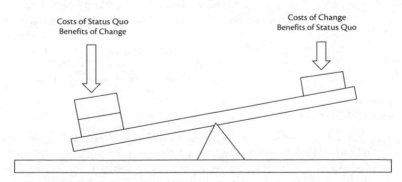

Figure 10.2. Decisional balance: weighing the costs and benefits. Reproduced with permission of Guilford Press. From Miller WR, and Rollnick S. *Motivational interviewing: preparing people for change.* Second edition. New York, Guilford Press, 2002, pp 15.

Cons of not changing	Pros of not changing
Financial cost	Relationships that work
My therapist will want to finish therapy	Decreased emotional pain

Not changing is difficult

Change is difficult. If it were easy you would not be reading this book. On the other hand, as you are probably aware, not changing is also difficult and perhaps even more difficult. Change by definition requires that we learn new behaviours and also let go of long-standing patterns of behaviour. These patterns are familiar and have been the best possible way we have found to get through our lives. To learn new ways and to let go of these old patterns is courageous.

 Comment from Wendy

For me, the decision to try or not try changing was agonizing—I felt like my insides were being torn apart. On one hand, the life I was living was excruciatingly painful, so I obviously desperately wanted to change. On the other hand, I could not picture a life for myself that I wanted and thought was possible, so what was the point of trying. I also knew that if I ever recovered that I would lose the mental health clinicians who were some of the very few people in my life. (As it happened, once I recovered there came a time when attending therapy was getting in the way of my life—a pretty good place to be in). In the end, I decided to give change a try. I did not want to fail, so deliberately approached change with small steps and just one step at a time. Nevertheless, I still had very disappointing setbacks; however, I was moving forward. And many small steps later I am where I am today. I am delighted and so relieved that somehow I decided on changing—yes, it wasn't always easy, but it was certainly well worth the effort.

Commitment

As change will be hard work requiring effort, it is important that you prepare yourself and make as big a commitment to change as you are able, while also compassionately giving yourself permission to make a small commitment that will be a start. Making realistic commitments to change tends to help people change. Commitments might include not giving up, seeking out therapy, or regularly attending therapy. Commitment to change is something that you will have to reassess continually throughout your recovery. Because change is hard, it is likely that part of you might want to give up on change from time to time. For this reason we encourage you to keep renewing your commitment to change, reminding yourself of the reasons why, on balance, the pros of change outweigh the cons.

Characteristics of people who change

1. Gap between where they are now and where they want to be.

2. Know where or how they can acquire skills required for change.

We are assuming that if you are reading this book you are doing so because there is a gap between where you are now and where you want to be and that you want to change so that things can be better. We are also assuming that if you confidently knew how to achieve these changes you would not be reading this book. Much of the rest of the book will focus on therapy as a place where you can obtain the skills required for change; however, first, you need to acquire or firm up your confidence that change is realistically possible for you.

Hope: acquiring confidence that change is realistically possible for you

There are a number of different ways that you can acquire confidence that change is possible and we encourage you to use whatever is going to be helpful for you. Some of you might be influenced by the scientific research showing that people with BPD can and do change. Some of you might find Wendy's story of recovery inspiring. Some of you might find it helpful to reflect upon positive changes that you have made in your lifetime, however small. This will provide hope for some of you that *you* can change. Some of you might find hope from witnessing friends or family members change. Some of you might find hope in your religious or spiritual beliefs. Many of you have already found hope or will find hope in engaging with a therapist. Some of you might be assisted by having a therapist who consistently holds the hope for you until such time as you can consistently hold it for yourself.

> Hope is looking 'for a favourable outcome within the realm of possibilities'
> Clarke (2003)

If you have the condition of BPD, the chances are that you will have had periods (maybe extensive) when you have been depressed, demoralized, and losing hope. Do we (Roy and Wendy) ever give up hope? There have been times when parts of ourselves have been despairing; however, this has always been both a temporary state and set in and surrounded in a larger foundation of hope. On these occasions hope has always re-emerged from the background to the foreground. On a few occasions we have been surprised at the unexpected places from which hope has arisen. These personal experiences support our position of not giving up. Hope in itself in not a guarantee of change; however, having hope has been shown to be associated with positive psychological outcomes. Because having hope is effective, it is important that we all work hard on creating the opportunities for hope to arise.

When we start on a journey to change we may unrealistically expect ourselves to develop new skills and drop all our old ways of coping *immediately*. Take change in small steps and practise these steps—practise does not make perfect, but it does improve skills. Don't give up. It took a long time to become the person that you are and it will take time to make robust lasting changes.

If you are taking a break from the journey of change and recovery, that is also fine. We all need breaks from trying hard for short periods. However, if you remain sufficiently distressed, you will need to keep the break from change fairly short and you might need to plan what you need to do to get back on the journey and when you are going to get back on the journey. Having a life that is satisfying is a truly wonderful thing.

> Don't give up!

- **Consciousness-raising.** Get informed about your condition and identify behaviours you want to change. This will help you in the contemplation stage.

- **Emotional arousal.** Focus on the gap between where you are and where you want to be. This can serve as the energy source to power your change, provided you have a pathway that you believe in that will assist you learning the skills you will require. Be sure to do this with compassion for yourself—do not give yourself a hard time for not being where you want to be.

- **Self-re-evaluation.** This can lead to recognition that you are not where you want to be. It will also require an awareness of what will be required of yourself (e.g. energy, time) and an awareness of what you will need to give up (e.g. alcohol) to change. You will be aware that change requires effort and you will have given up on the magical effortless pathway to recovery that we all would like but that can be so counter-productive.

- **Helping relationships.** These can support and encourage you and assist your learning of new skills required for change.

- **Commitment.** Set in place your plan for your recovery, take the first small step and be realistic. Commitment to change is courageous. Pat yourself on the back and make a commitment to re-commit again and again and again throughout your recovery, especially when things get really hard.

- **Countering.** This refers to putting in place new healthy behaviours and thoughts to replace behaviours and thoughts that you have identified as problems. For example, this may be exercising if you are depressed and inactive or self-talk that you are a human being with rights if you have a tendency to be overly submissive or harsh with yourself.

- **Environment control.** This involves reorganizing what you can in your environment that will promote your achieving your goals (e.g. avoiding bars if you have a drinking problem, going to social events if you are lonely). It may be getting assistance from people in your community to help you change by rewarding you for skilful action and to not reward you for unskilful action.

◆ **Reward.** This has been shown to be one of the most effective means of creating change. In the beginning, reward yourself at every opportunity for every positive step that you take. Rewards can include praising yourself for your efforts or a reward such as going to the movies or a meal at a café—whatever is the kind of thing you enjoy. Later on as you build successes, you can stretch out the interval between rewards, but early in the change process, reward yourself at every opportunity.

 Comment from Wendy

It is now 7 years since I met diagnostic criteria for BPD. I am now living a life again. After many years on a benefit I am working and have an active family and social life. My life is not perfect but is definitely satisfying, filled as it is with plenty of pleasure, meaning, and purpose.

Elements associated with change

As a guide for putting in place the things you need to change it might be helpful to consider the elements found by Prochaska *et al.* (1994) to be associated with the process of change and for you to consider how you can increase the likelihood of positive change.

 Comment from Wendy

I found small rewards worked really well for me—I started out by rewarding myself for tidying one room of the house by something delicious to eat at home. Later I would reward myself for going out of the house by treating myself to a coffee at a specialty coffee café. Eventually I got to the point of rewarding myself for going to work, by buying a luxury each payday. After a while the natural rewards of recovery themselves were more than enough on their own, and there was no need actively to reward myself beyond this. I still sometimes treat myself, simply because I like treating myself.

Making change work: our suggestions

Identify problems and reasons for change

It is very hard for us to change something until we know what the problem is. Becoming aware of the problem is an important first step to change. Developing a personal belief of the value of change and making this a priority in your life will also go a long way to sustain you when things get tough. We encourage you to write down your reasons for changing as this can have a solidifying effect. As you no doubt are aware, there is no 'magic wand' to wave in your recovery, nor is there a magically right moment to wait for change. As change is difficult, we encourage you to be your own cheerleader, telling and re-telling yourself why you need to change.

Set small realistic goals

Gather the information that you need to know that will assist you in changing. We find it helpful to define goals in terms of specific behaviours (e.g. enrolling in study, visiting friends) rather than emotions (e.g. feel happier). Plan and prepare for your recovery—try avoiding acting impulsively. It is important to take a first small step. Set realistic expectations of yourself. This way you can build up small successes.

Explore solutions to anxiety about change

Any anxiety that you have about change needs to be attended to, including talking to your therapist. Some people are anxious that positive change will result in people withdrawing their support, including their therapist. If this is the case, you will need to discuss this with the relevant people to ensure that this anxiety does not hold you back from change. Like many people with BPD, you may want to change but also find change daunting. For this reason it is important that you and your therapist respectfully explore expectations of the rate of change. Setting your expectations for change too low might result in a therapy that is stuck, not going anywhere. On the other hand, setting your expectations for change too high might be overly daunting and work against you, actually resulting in less change.

❓ Key questions to ask yourself about change

How will I benefit if I change?

_____

_____

_____

_____

What are the positive things about change?

_____

_____

_____

_____

What are the negative things about change?

_____

_____

_____

_____

What will happen if I change?

_____

_____

_____

_____

Are there things about change that I am concerned about?

_____

_____

_____

_____

Is change important?

_____

_____

Is change important now?

_____

_____

What do I need to do to find hope that change is possible?

_____

_____

_____

_____

What do I need to do to maintain hope that change is possible?

_____

_____

_____

_____

What do I need to do to give me more confidence that I can change?

_____

_____

_____

_____

Do I need more information on BPD?

_____

_____

Do I need more information about therapy options?

_____

_____

Am I asking the right questions to get the information I need?

_____

_____

What do I need to do to acquire the necessary skills to change?

_____

_____

_____

_____

Do I need a professional to explain to me how I can learn the skills I need
for change?

_____

_____

What can I learn from my past successful efforts at change?

_____

_____

_____

_____

What can I learn from my past unsuccessful efforts at change?

_____

_____

_____

_____

What, if anything, is holding me back from change?

_____

_____

_____

_____

What are going to be barriers in my environment to change?

_____

_____

_____

_____

What are going to be my internal barriers to change?

_____

_____

_____

_____

What is the next step I need to take towards change?

_____

_____

What do I need to take the next step towards change?

_____

_____

_____

_____

I plan to take the following specific actions:

	When?
_____	When?
_____	When?
_____	When?
_____	When?
_____	When?
_____	When?
_____	When?
_____	When?
_____	When?
_____	When?

Prepare your support people to support you and you to support them

Clarify who the people are who will support you through your times of change. This may include family, friends, and professionals. Having people to support you will make the hard job of change a little easier. As well as setting up your support system to support, encourage, and cheerlead you to change, it can also be helpful that others are prepared to tell you what an amazing job you have done after you have made changes, however small. In this way you will more probably be energized to continue the hard work of change. Scientific research has shown that rewards and praise are a far more productive means of supporting change than scolding. You in turn will need to reward rather than scold them for all the things that they do to help you. You might also need to advise people of the limits and boundaries of what you can do for them and they might likewise need to advise you of the limits and boundaries of what they can do for you. In this way you support others to support you.

If you have decided on a next step, congratulate yourself on taking the next step. If you are not ready to take the next step, compassionately accept where you are at, without giving yourself a hard time.

11

Psychological treatments

 Key points

- Cognitive-behavioural therapy refers to therapies that focus on cognitions (thinking) and behaviours.

- Dialectical behaviour therapy is a cognitive-behavioural therapy especially well suited for treating people with BPD. Standard dialectical behaviour therapy involves individual therapy, telephone calls, and skills training.

- STEPPS teaches structured cognitive-behavioural skills as a value-added programme to existing treatment. Key professionals, family, and friends learn to reinforce effective skills taught, providing a reinforcing community.

- Schema-focused therapy has cognitive therapy at its core. Four dominant shifting dimensions of the client are identified, each having an associated structured treatment strategy.

- Cognitive analytical therapy is derived from a combination of cognitive therapy and psychoanalytical* therapy and is generally a brief therapy of 16–40 sessions.

- Mentalizing* refers to the capacity to know and experience the psychological world of ourselves/others seeking to understand/know mental states underlying behaviour.

- In psychodynamic*/psychoanalytical* therapy, the relationship between you and your therapist is the central and essential ingredient for change.

- Supportive psychotherapy uses the 'real' positive relationship between your therapist and yourself as a means of focusing on your day to day issues.

- 'Case management' (sic) focuses on common sense practical day to day issues utilizing whatever resources are available including community-based resources. In some services 'case management' (sic) refers more specifically to tasks associated with money, benefits, housing, food, and legal issues.

- High-quality standard treatment will be provided by an individual or organization that has developed a way of thinking about and treating people like yourself with BPD based on significant experience.

In this section, we have used the language professionals use to label their treatments. Do not despair if the words in this paragraph are unknown to you—you will be in good company. The rest of this chapter will describe what these words mean. The following descriptions of treatments start with the behaviourally dominant dialectical behaviour therapy (DBT) and STEPPS treatments, followed by the cognitively dominant schema-focused therapy, then cognitive-behavioural therapy moving to the integrative cognitive analytical therapy and then onto the psychodynamically based mentalization*, then psychodynamic*/psychoanalytical* therapy, and finishing with supportive psychotherapy, 'case management' and high-quality standard treatment.

Dialectical behaviour therapy

DBT is a cognitive-behavioural therapy (see below) that is especially well suited to treating people with BPD. The first time we came across the word 'dialectical' we had to run for the dictionary. Dialectics refers to bringing together (synthesizing) apparently conflicting positions such as liking a person while at the same time disliking some things about them. The central dialectic in DBT is for you and your clinician to get the balance right between accepting yourself just as you are and engaging in efforts to change. DBT can be provided in many different settings with a degree of flexibility while remaining true to the treatment. Prior to beginning treatment you will be involved in discussions clarifying common specific goals (e.g. decreasing self-harm urges) that you and your therapist will work on, orientating you to treatment and discussions that might build your motivation for change and help you make a commitment to the therapy. Standard DBT involves three components; individual therapy, telephone calls, and skills training.

Individual therapy focuses on understanding how your behaviours make sense (your best way of coping that you currently know) and affirming your struggles. You and your individual therapist will explore problem behaviours (e.g. urges to self-harm) and then healthy solutions to these problems via the use of problem and solution analysis described later in Section 3.

Depending on your therapist and treating organization, you might be encouraged to make brief telephone calls at times of distress to receive skills coaching so that you can get through the crisis without making things worse.

Skills training usually takes place in a group but can be taught individually. Skills training teaches skills that help you strengthen and use existing skills across a range of situations and learn new skills of living. Distress tolerance skills are, as the name suggests, skills to help you get through distressing times without making things worse. Interpersonal effectiveness skills are, as the name indicates, skills that help you with relationships. This will involve assertiveness skills while also paying attention to your relationships and to your own self-respect. Emotion regulation skills assist you to feel your emotions early on when they are manageable, thereby decreasing problem behaviours associated with overwhelmingly intense emotions or problems associated with numbing out. Emotion regulation skills also teach you how to develop a state that decreases your vulnerability to distressing emotions and how to decrease distressing emotions when faced with a cue that previously would have resulted in distress. Emotion regulation as well as teaching how to accept emotions as they are also involves learning how to generate desired emotions deliberately. Mindfulness skills are attention control skills that help with the effectiveness of all the other skills and with problem and solution analysis, and are described further in Section 3.

The relationship between you and your therapist is critical and will need to be talked about when problems arise as they invariably will during treatment. It will be important that you feel heard, understood, and validated by your therapist for who you are. The therapy relationship serves then as a method through which behaviour therapy (problem and solution analysis and skills training) can take place.

STEPPS

STEPPS stands for Systems Training for Emotional Predictability and Problem Solving and teaches structured cognitive-behavioural skills to the person with BPD in a weekly skills group over 20 weeks followed by a monthly advanced skills group. STEPPS is not intended as a stand alone complete treatment but rather as a value-added programme improving existing treatment and possibly decreasing the frequency of need for existing treatments. Educational information about BPD (alternatively referred to as emotional intensity disorder) is taught providing a common compassionate and effective way of understanding BPD. This is followed by the teaching of effective emotion and behaviour skills to deal with emotional intensity to both clients and their family/friends. Key professionals, family, and friends learn to reinforce effective skills taught, providing a reinforcing community. STEPPS expects that clients will take a responsible role in helping their relevant community to be an effective reinforcing community for them, reinforcing healthy productive behaviours.

Schema-focused therapy

Schema-focused therapy is an integrative therapy with cognitive therapy (see below) at its core. Four dominant shifting parts of the client are identified, with each part having a related structured treatment strategy for both the therapist and client.

1. The 'abandoned child' aspect requires the therapist to empathize with the client and for the client to nurture themselves.

2. The 'angry child' aspect requires the therapist to express empathy balanced with appropriate reality testing and the client to find healthy ways of expressing anger.

3. The 'punitive parent' aspect refers to that part of the client that is self-critical and requires the therapist to assist the client to fight off and get rid of the 'punitive parent' aspect.

4. The 'detached protector' refers to that part of the client that is emotionally detached to protect against excessive pain. The 'detached protector' aspect needs reassurance from the therapist and the client that it is OK to feel emotions. This can be done by timely exploration of painful memories and by dealing with the 'abandoned, angry, and punitive child' aspects.

Cognitive-behavioural therapy

Cognitive-behavioural therapy refers to therapies that focus on cognitions (thinking) and behaviours.

A common language description of cognitions is the term 'self-talk'. These are the things we tell ourselves that can either improve the situation or cause it to deteriorate. An example of productive self-talk if you are in DBT is the assumption that 'I am doing the best that I know how and I want to do better'. If you are anxious you might try using self-talk such as 'I am anxious and I have got through it before'. Cognitive therapy will encourage you to name thoughts as thoughts and not facts. This might result in a change from, 'I am totally useless' to, 'I am having a thought that I am totally useless'. This allows room to explore the chances that our negative thoughts might not be facts. Cognitive therapy might also explore the evidence for whether our beliefs are accurate or inaccurate. If the evidence does not support our beliefs (e.g. nobody is 'totally' useless), then therapy will explore alternative more effective self-talk (e.g. 'I am skilful and effective at many activities and have yet to develop other skills').

Behaviour therapy will explore problems and behaviours that you want to work on, seeking to understand these behaviours and why they occur, followed by working together on solutions you can put into place. Standard behavioural treatment for depression, for example, will encourage you in maintaining your activity level as much as possible and doing things that are pleasurable, purposeful, or meaningful. Behaviour therapy for anxiety will involve your developing, with your therapist, a graded hierarchy (ladder) of situations where, in small graded steps, you can 'expose' yourself to what you are anxious about while finding ways of keeping your anxiety at reasonable levels. In this way you can build up successes, and the feared situations become less fearful. Whatever your biggest problems are, engaging in regular activities (behaviours) that you are competent at will build and maintain your sense of mastery, competence, and self-worth.

Cognitive analytical therapy

This therapy is a combination of cognitive therapy and psychoanalytical therapy, and is generally a brief therapy of 16–40 sessions. You will share your life story or what is called 'narrative', after which your therapist will write you a letter that they will read out aloud to you. This letter, called a 'reformulation', describes the important patterns of your life and relationships. A diagram is made of these patterns that also identify 'snags' or barriers to your recovery that will need to be overcome. Hearing the reformulation letter will hopefully leave you feeing well understood, and along with the diagram, with specific tangible means of changing your life patterns and rewriting your life story. Therapy will explore how you might be able to overcome the past patterns with new strategies called 'exits'. At the end of therapy both you and your therapist will write each other a letter summarizing your journey in therapy in a manner intended to support your efforts after treatment concludes.

Mentalization*-based therapy

Mentalization* refers to the capacity to know and experience the psychological world of ourselves and, as best as we are able, the psychological world of others. This includes seeing our world viewed from outside of ourselves as others see us, and seeing the world of others viewed from inside themselves. Mentalizing* also seeks to understand and know the mental states underlying behaviour. Mentalizing* is the capacity to know and use our minds to the best effect.

As human beings our capacity to mentalize* is interfered with by overwhelming emotions such as agonizing anxiety or anger, or being overwhelmingly in love. When in these states we might 'lose our minds' so to speak and act 'mindlessly'. After the event, we might describe ourselves as having 'lost the plot' or 'I must have been out of my mind'. Mentalization*-based therapy will aim to increase our capacity to not 'lose our minds' when experiencing intense emotions but to remain mindful of ourselves and others—that is mentalizing*.

Mentalization*-based therapy will focus discussion on how we can improve our ability for psychological experiencing and psychological consideration. Life situations and relationships including the therapy relationship are all used to encourage getting into our minds skilfully. The focus is on the here and now of our minds. Practising mentalizing will result in a growing psychological self-awareness that will empower us to attend skilfully to life situations using all of our growing psychological skills. Mentalizing* practice will also increase our awareness of the psychological world of others so essential for effective interpersonal relationships.

Mentalization*-based therapy highly values the critical importance of a stable secure valued relationship between client and therapist that will provide a psychologically secure base to explore and practise mentalizing*. If our childhoods were filled with overwhelming emotions we will not have had the necessary opportunities to practise and learn mentalizing*, so necessary for adult functioning. The therapy relationship serves to correct this by providing an environment where we can feel safe enough, and not be overwhelmed by emotions thereby assisting our capacity to practise mentalizing*.

Further related information can be found in Chapter 26 ('Self-reflection') in Section 3.

Psychodynamic*/psychoanalytical* psychotherapy

In psychodynamic*/psychoanalytical* therapy, the relationship between you and your therapist is the central and essential ingredient for change. You and your therapist will work at developing a relationship where you can feel that the therapy time is your time dedicated to you and your goals. The task in therapy will be for you and your therapist to 'bring to light of day' behaviours, thoughts, and emotions that can assist you achieving your goals. This self-reflection is discussed in Section 3.

You and your therapist will aim to reach a position where you feel understood; feeling the empathy of your therapist. Inevitably there will be times when you will not feel your therapist's empathy. At these times your and your therapist's task is to get this difference of understanding back on track and also to come to terms with the fact that your therapist will not be perfectly empathic but hopefully will be seen by you as 'good enough'. This process might help you with your 'all or nothing', black and white thinking as you begin, within the therapy relationship, to bring together the strengths and weaknesses of your therapist, yourself, and the world in general.

The goal of therapy is that once you experience the relationship as safe, caring, and empathic you will begin to explore who you are and how you want to be in the relationship. Through this self-reflective process you will develop a growing sense of who you are. Being who you are in the presence of somebody who is safe, caring, and empathic is likely to help you view yourself as likeable and of worth and value. Your self-worth and self-esteem will grow out of this warm, safe, attached relationship, with your therapist leaving you well placed for successful relationships and for achieving your goals.

It is possible that you will feel about and relate to your therapist the way that you have related to other people in your life or how you would have liked to have related to people in the past (e.g. a parent who was not there). This is referred to technically as transference and will be a focus of attention for some psychodynamic*/psychoanalytical* therapists. Transference refers to the transferring of feelings that belong in the past to people in the present. We all do this to some degree. For example, when people talk of someone having a 'chip on his/her shoulder' they are implying that the person is relating in the present in the manner they do because of past experiences. Understanding and reflecting upon your past and current patterns of behaviour and relating can be used by yourself in your therapy as an opportunity to develop constructive patterns of relating, making changes that are consistent with your goals.

Supportive psychotherapy

Supportive psychotherapy uses the 'real' (as opposed to transference) positive relationship between your therapist and yourself as a means of focusing on your day to day realities. Your past will not be explored as a major part of your therapy and your therapy will be practical and matter-of-fact, focusing on common sense issues. Cognitive-behavioural therapy methods, education, skills training, advice, empathy, support, and encouragement will be used flexibly as necessary. Frequency and duration of contact will be flexible and dependent on your needs. It will be expected that change will flow out of a positive respectful relationship where your skills and courage will be celebrated.

Milton and Banfai (1999) write that for generalist clinicians who do not view themselves as therapists and are not trained in a specific model:

> ... a supportive psychotherapy is probably the easiest to maintain, allowing for a workable combination of different interventions within a coherent model of care. In this way of working, the clinician acts as a secure base, strengthening the client's adaptive functioning through suggestion, education, limit setting and facilitating therapeutic alliance. Creation of the alliance over the long term, coupled with consistency and availability, may be of greater importance to success with the client than any of the specific therapeutic interventions themselves.

A supportive psychotherapy can mesh rather well with a 'case management' (sic) approach.

'Case management' (sic)

This might be a term used to describe the type of treatment you are receiving. We are in agreement with people with BPD who state that they are not 'cases' to be 'managed' but people to be treated. However, we have used the word 'case management' (sic) in the event that this term is used to describe your treatment. An alternative term could be 'recovery co-ordination'. The term 'case management' is well established in many systems and in no way do we suggest that receiving a 'case management' approach will be unhelpful, or that the people providing 'case management' have unhelpful attitudes, merely that, in our opinion, the wording is less than ideal. 'Case management' can be very helpful in assisting you on your road to recovery.

'Case management' (sic) usually refers to a treatment provided by a person who does not consider themselves a therapist or is not in the role of therapist. It is a term often used to describe the treatment relationship where treatment is provided within an organization. The person carrying out the treatment might be a nurse, psychologist, psychiatrist, social worker, occupational therapist, 'case manager' (sic), or service co-ordinator. The 'case management' (sic) work might be integrated with other treatment such as therapy, medication, supportive accommodation, hospital, and crisis treatments.

'Case management' (sic) may have significant similarities to supportive psychotherapy (see above), focusing on common sense practical day to day issues and utilizing whatever resources are available including community-based resources. Your 'case manager' (sic) will have the task of working with you (collaboratively) to develop and maintain a treatment plan that includes and brings together all relevant treatment providers. This might include establishing goals and monitoring treatment. In some services 'case management' (sic) refers more specifically to tasks associated with money and state benefits, finding and maintaining appropriate housing, adequate food, and various legal issues.

High-quality standard treatment

High-quality standard treatment will be provided by an individual or organization that has developed a way of thinking about and treating people like yourself with BPD based on significant experience. Organizations will have clear policies, procedures, and guidelines that will guide your treatment. Quality supervision will be available to the therapist who is treating you. Your therapist will have interest and experience in treating people like yourself with BPD. In organizations, your therapy will be supported by hospital, crisis, and medication treatments as applicable. Your therapist will use skills that they are familiar with and might draw from cognitive-behavioural therapy, DBT, cognitive analytical therapy, psychodynamic*/psychoanalytical* therapy, mentalization*, supportive therapy, and 'case management' (sic).

Similarities across different treatment models

All models value the relationship that you have with your therapist as essential for effective treatment. All models have expectations and roles clearly defined, including a considered response to crises that will be effective in helping you achieve your goals. As well as recognizing and empathizing with your difficulties, all models will emphasize your skills and strengths so that your abilities can be valued and grown. All models, to the best of our knowledge, will encourage self-awareness via your formal or informal self-reflection as a guiding influence on identifying problems and solutions to your problems. Clinicians working in all models will need to be well grounded in the model of treatment that they are using.

Complementary nature of different treatment models

Different models can be used skilfully to complement one another. For example, medication and 'case management' (sic) might complement a DBT, cognitive-behavioural therapy, cognitive analytical, or psychodynamic* psychotherapy. However, it will be important that you and your treating clinicians ensure that different treatment approaches are pulling in the same general direction.

12

What to expect from treatment

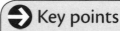Key points

♦ Treatment for BPD is generally a relatively long-term commitment, both on your part, and the part of your clinicians.

♦ The average frequency of therapy sessions if you are seeing a therapist might be one hour/week, with some people being seen more often and some less often.

♦ Change is a process that does not work in a straight line, so do not be disappointed if you feel like you are taking two steps forward and one back.

♦ From every clinician you should expect respect, clear limits/boundaries, knowledge, hope, a relatively long-term view, collaboration, and confidentiality.

♦ If you have been in the mental health system for a long time and have only recently been given a BPD diagnosis, do not despair, this could represent a major turning point in your recovery.

Duration of treatment

Treatment for BPD is generally a relatively long-term commitment, both on your part, and the part of your clinicians. Provided it is what you want, effective treatment will generally be for a minimum of a year and may appropriately take several years. All the evidence-based psychotherapies have lasted at least one year and have been restricted to this time due to research constraints rather than clinical optimum, which would in most situations be longer than this.

The amount of time you are in therapy will depend on internal and external factors. Internal factors will include the problems, goals, and skills you have prior to entering treatment, and your stage of change. External factors will be the availability of relevant treatment options including the amount of treatment an insurance company or public mental health service is able to provide.

Provided relevant treatment is available to you, we encourage you to be compassionate on yourself regarding how long treatment is taking provided treatment is productive, heading in the desired directions, and treatment goals are being met. Resolving difficulties in a safe manner can be a lengthy process. So long as you are doing your best and progress is being made, do not give yourself a hard time for how long therapy takes.

Amount of treatment

The average frequency of therapy sessions if you are seeing a therapist might be one hour/week, with some people being seen more often and some less often. You may also attend a skills training group or therapy group, have some availability for crisis contact, and see a clinician who prescribes medication.

Two steps forward and one step back

Change is a process that does not work in a straight line, so do not be disappointed if you feel like you are taking two steps forward and one back. Keeping a journal of positive experiences and times you have successfully tried new skills and behaviours can be a useful tool to help you see the gains you are making when times are tough.

What you can expect from clinicians

As clinicians are all unique individuals, you will learn what you can rely on and expect from that individual. Broadly, however, there are certain behaviours and attitudes that are reasonable to expect from any clinician.

Respect

It is reasonable for you to expect to be listened to and treated with respect and dignity. This includes respecting your culture, religious beliefs, and sexual orientation. If you feel you are being treated disrespectfully, you should consider discussing your feelings with a view to improving the mutual respect between yourself and the other person. If this is not productive and you feel that you are being repeatedly treated disrespectfully, we encourage you to reflect whether your perceptions could be inaccurate and whether you have a role in contributing to the problem and address these if applicable. If you still believe that you are being treated disrespectfully and have explored all options with the person involved then you might need to consider the possibility of finding a different clinician.

Limits and boundaries

You can expect that your clinician will have and stick to professional and ethical boundaries that support your safe and effective treatment. These boundaries include it *never* being OK to have a sexual relationship with you. If this is happening, seek assistance from an advocate or someone you trust. Other boundaries include keeping to agreed upon length of appointments, agreed upon availability outside scheduled sessions, and sessions uninterrupted by telephone calls/pagers/cell phones except in emergencies. The same courtesy will be expected of you. Another limit/boundary that your clinician might have is shortening the session if you are intoxicated (alcohol or other drugs).

Knowledge

You can expect that your clinician will have the knowledge of somebody of their profession and will keep reasonably up to date with current thinking and practice.

Hope

You can expect that your therapist believes in your ability to recover and achieve a satisfying life. As discussed earlier, this is a realistic hope, and sometimes when you are struggling, the hope of the clinicians around you may be all you have to hang on to.

A long-term view

You can expect that your clinician/s will try hard to 'hold the big picture', especially at times when you are fighting to get through one moment at a time.

Collaboration

You can expect that your clinician/s will work closely with you and involve you, wherever possible, in all decisions about your care and treatment.

You can expect to work collaboratively wherever possible, with your clinicians to develop your treatment and crisis treatment plans. You may want to request having an input into notes written in your file.

Plan ahead for breaks in treatment

Therapists being away is a time of difficulty, well recognized by both therapists and clients with BPD. You can expect your therapist to plan ahead and give you as much warning as possible of any expected breaks in treatment (vacation, study, conferences, etc.) so that together you can develop strategies and plans for the period of their absence.

Privacy and confidentiality

Your clinician is bound by a professional code of ethics to maintain your confidentiality. You can expect that any information kept about you is kept securely, and many countries provide for your right to see this information if you request it through appropriate processes.

Different professions, countries, states, and localities may have different legislation about confidentiality. However, it is quite likely that exceptions to the confidentiality rule will be discussions with treating team, treating organization, clinical supervisor (good standard practice), court order (subpoena), and where there is significant risk to the safety of yourself or someone else. In the latter case your clinician is likely to have an obligation to inform relevant people.

If you have been in the mental health system for a long time and have only recently been given a BPD diagnosis

If this has been your experience, you might have been given numerous diagnoses and received and embarked on several treatments in the past. It might be that having gone back to yet another clinician and getting yet another diagnosis has left you understandably feeling demoralized. Assuming the BPD diagnosis is accurate, this could represent a major turning point in your recovery. This was certainly the situation for Wendy. Wendy had several previous diagnoses, and treatment was ineffective because she was receiving treatment for a condition she did not have. While initially demoralized about receiving a BPD diagnosis, this also represented a defining moment in Wendy's recovery as she could now engage in treatment appropriate to her condition. Hope was restored and ultimately treatment for BPD was effective.

13

First contact with health professionals

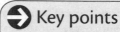
This chapter explores your first contact with health professionals. If you are already being seen by a health professional we encourage you nevertheless to read this chapter for the principles outlined. If you are making first contact with a therapist, there is likely to be information in this chapter that does apply to your situation.

Access

In most cases a health professional such as your family doctor can refer you to a mental health professional or service. Other people who may refer you are from hospital emergency departments, social services, and the police. It is generally better for you to make contact with the health professional or service prior to a crisis; however, be sure to make contact in a crisis for the first time if you need to. Many mental health services have an emergency or crisis number that you can contact in a crisis. If you have difficulty accessing mental health services, enlist the help of supportive family or friends. Finding out the required pathways to accessing mental health professionals and services can sometimes be tricky, so keep trying if you feel you need their help.

While things have improved dramatically regarding attitudes towards people with BPD, some areas, organizations, and clinicians continue to have a stigmatizing attitude and/or pessimistic view of treatment outcomes and/or are not well informed about treatment options and skills required. Readers need to be aware of this potential stigma, misinformation, and lack of information among the clinical community. If you can access the organization's and clinician's perceptions about BPD before the first session this would be a plus. Some clinicians do not have a stigmatizing attitude but choose not to treat people with BPD. This position is honest and open, and quite acceptable in our opinion, provided that any organization that is responsible for treating all mental health disorders in the community has willing clinicians available to treat people with BPD. It is our opinion that it is unacceptable for organizations who are mandated to provide mental health treatment for a community to not treat people with BPD but treat people with other mental health conditions such as schizophrenia* and bipolar affective disorder*. The importance of seeking out a clinician who understands BPD and believes in recovery can't be stressed enough.

Getting familiar with available services

Mental health services might have an information pack that describes what services are available and who the professional/s are.

Most treatment for BPD takes place in the community. A few residential therapy centres exist but these are becoming more uncommon nowadays. You can expect almost all professionals and services to have some arrangements for crisis contact outside of scheduled therapy hours, should the need arise. Make sure you understand these crisis arrangements. Public service community mental health centres are often made up of teams of nurses, psychologists, social workers, occupational therapists, counsellors, therapists, and psychiatrists who will schedule times to see you at the centre. Inpatient psychiatric hospital units are a possibility at times of acute crisis. Some areas have specialist services for clients with BPD and for clients from different age and cultural groups. Some professionals in private practice will specialize in BPD or working with people of specific ages (e.g. youth) or cultural background

Taking or not taking a support person

For some of you, taking a support person with you to your first appointment can be helpful. This person might help you stay focused on your goals and needs, ask questions you intended to ask but forget, and be another pair of ears so that you can check out with them what was said later. For others of you, taking a support person could be unhelpful as they might get in the way, confuse the picture, or shift the focus to their agenda.

Feelings about the first appointment

When you see a professional for the first time, you may have feelings of hopeful anticipation that someone may be able to help. On the other hand, it is quite possible that your feelings may be in turmoil. It is common to feel overwhelmed and scared. Another common experience is feeling ashamed that you need help. There is no need to feel shameful about seeking out assistance from a professional. BPD is a recognized legitimate condition that seriously affects people's lives, including probably yours. If you could have solved your problems yourself you would have, and professionals are trained to help people like yourself. You have the same right to treatment as somebody whose life is seriously affected by physical illness. Seeking out treatment might be one of the most skilful actions that you undertake. Acknowledging a problem and committing yourself to change is a courageous step that we applaud. We encourage you to give yourself a pat on the back.

Information gathering and giving at the first session

When you first have contact with a health professional, the professional will make connection with you and assess your needs and difficulties. This usually involves lots of questions. Because BPD affects most areas of your life, questions about your whole life are likely to be necessary. Do your best to answer these questions openly, being as clear as you are able about your difficulties and needs. There may well be some details of your life that might be appropriate to keep to yourself until such time as you get to know the professional better. An example is that while it will be helpful for the professional to know if you have had a past history of sexual abuse, it may be appropriate that you do not talk about the full details of this until you feel that you know the professional well enough to feel safe sharing this material. The professional may also request your permission to source further information from the person who referred you or from family and friends.

Sometimes sharing information about yourself in a first session can lead to a strong emotional reaction. Some people deal with this by choosing to have the most important points of their history written down to give to the clinician they will be meeting. If you do this be sure to be precise and focused and provide information that is brief. We would suggest no longer than two typed A4 pages long. This might save you the experience of feeling grilled and interrogated.

Be clear and direct

Try to be clear about the role of the person you are speaking with and ways in which they may be able to assist you. You may need to tell the professional that being in control is important to you, and that you want to be fully involved in all decisions about your care and treatment. If it is what you want, you may state that you want a support person to be involved in major decisions about treatment.

Remember, clinicians are not mind readers and are not going to be able to guess your wishes. You will have to tell them. Be clear and direct about what you believe will help and what you believe will not, and the reasons why. Finally, if you are struggling to find the words to express what you want to say or to answer a question, say so. This will encourage clearer understanding between you and the professional.

 Comment from Wendy

One of my downfalls was worrying that representing myself accurately or assertively making requests would lead to my being turned down and I would feel rejected. I was sad and disappointed for a long time that health professionals did not read my mind and respond to my unspoken needs, resulting in me feeling devastated and alone. Eventually, as I learned to trust my judgements of people more, I learned to be clear and direct with the people I trusted about how I was feeling and what I needed, and, to my pleasure, many more of my needs were met. Some people were less responsive when I shared how I was feeling and asserted myself and I had to distinguish between these people and those with whom more open sharing was wise.

Don't be afraid to ask questions

Don't be afraid to ask questions or pick up brochures about what the professional or service offers. Keep asking and discussing if you do not understand the answer. Many people working in the BPD area unintentionally use jargon. We may have got used to the language that we use among ourselves, forgetting that this is not the language of everyday people. If you do not understand, neither will most of the population—there is no need to feel embarrassed or ashamed—simply ask for clarification—assertively and respectfully.

Wrapping up the first session

Some services will have you seen initially by a person whose sole job is to see you once so that they can make a referral for you to see the person who is most likely to be of assistance. If this is the case, knowing that the assessing clinician will see you just the once will help you have realistic expectations of them and the session. The assessing clinician may offer to provide treatment themselves or may refer you on to another member of their team. If you are being referred to another service or clinician, be sure you understand why the professional believes this to be in your best interest, so that you reduce the risk of feeling rejected, which most people with BPD are exquisitely sensitive to.

For many of you, your first contact with mental health services may have been at a time of crisis, when you were least prepared to deal with the complexities involved. Our advice to you is to take charge of your role in your treatment from now on, maximizing the likelihood of the treatment working for you.

> **Explore how you can take charge of your recovery**

14

Choosing a therapist (where such a choice exists)

 Key points

♦ Choosing a therapist is one of the most important things you will do on your recovery journey.

♦ The factor we think that you should give greatest priority to in selecting a therapist is therapeutic competence in working with people with BPD.

♦ Consider preparing for your first face-to-face meeting by writing down or highlighting the key points you want to know.

Who is available?

If you believe that you have BPD, we strongly encourage you to seek out a therapist if you do not already have one, as the research evidence is that this is generally the most important dimension of recovery. If you are receiving treatment from a public mental health service, or funded through insurance, there may be some restrictions on who is available to you. If your choice is restricted you will have to make the best of what is available to you or, where this is clearly not working, make a case to the relevant organization for increased flexibility. The case you make will need to demonstrate that increased choice will improve your and the relevant organization's goals.

Where to start?

If you have never consulted a therapist before, you may not know where to begin. A good place to start is by carefully going over Chapter 11 on 'Psychological treatments', assessing which type of therapy feels best for you. You might want to develop a small list of possible therapists from insurers, the telephone directory, Citizens Advice Bureau, your GP, and anyone you know who is receiving treatment for similar problems for their recommendations.

Professional's background

You will note that therapists usually have letters of qualifications after their names (e.g. MA, MS, MSW, PhD, PsyD, MD, RPN). Most therapists will have a basic qualification in a field of mental health. Common base qualifications are those of psychology, psychiatry, social work, psychotherapy, counselling, and medicine. Many of these professionals will then complete a higher level qualification, with what is referred to as a master's qualification, or a higher level again referred to as a doctorate. Following their successful training, the therapist will almost always and in our opinion should always be a member of a professional organization that will have a professional code of ethics, minimal standards, and mechanisms in place to promote competence. This professional organization will usually provide the therapist with an annual practicing certificate subject to the therapist meeting certain annual standards such as adequate supervision and ongoing education.

Therapist competence, and gender, age, and culture

Another point to consider is the gender of the therapist. Assess whether the gender of the therapist is a significant issue for you. For example, a woman who was sexually abused by a male may decide she feels more comfortable working with a woman therapist. You may have a preference for the age group of the therapist. You may prefer working with somebody close to your own age, whom you feel can identify with the issues of your age group or you may prefer someone older or younger. You may wish to choose a therapist with a similar life view or religious affiliation to yourself, especially if you wish to incorporate aspects of this life view into your therapy, such as prayer for example.

Competence as a therapist generally does not necessarily mean competence in working with people with BPD. Many people will be excellent and experienced therapists, who come highly recommended, but who may specialize in treating people with anxiety or depression, for example, and have had little experience or success working with people with BPD. Experience working with people with BPD is certainly to be highly valued.

Finding the right clinician can involve asking questions about the clinician's experience, training, and education in treating BPD, and learning what type of therapy they believe works best for people with BPD. These questions will save you a lot of time and allow you to have reasonable control of decisions about choosing a therapist.

At the end of the day, the factor we think that you should give greatest priority to in selecting a therapist is therapeutic competence in working with people with BPD. If, in addition to this you are able to select a therapist with other factors that suit you, such as age and gender, then do so. We do not, however, believe that you should place factors such as age and gender above competence in working with people with BPD.

Initial phone call

Where you have some choice of therapist, once you have a small list of names with qualifications and credentials you are happy with, you can begin to narrow the list down. A phone call to each person on your list is a good way to start. You will need to use all of your interpersonal skills. First, ask the therapist if they would be willing to spend a few minutes talking about the possibility of therapy and thanking them for their willingness to do so. Indicate to the therapist that the questions you are asking are about getting treatment set up on the right footing. Finish by thanking them for their time.

If the person you are calling is the person that you want to end up working with, you will need to do everything you can to make the therapist want to work with you. (There is no point in you wanting to work with a therapist who does not want to work with you.) This will involve being as clear as you can of your objectives in making the call, being respectful and thanking the person at the beginning and at the end of the call.

Example

Hello my name is . . . I am calling about the possibility of engaging in therapy with you. I have a few things I would like to ask and discuss. Is now a good time or would it be more convenient for you to call me back later? Now is OK—oh good, thank you for your time. I recognize that therapy is a big commitment, so wanted to ask a few things so as to set up therapy on the right note.

You might be anxious about making the call or get anxious during the call. Highlighting or writing down the questions beforehand that you plan to ask is likely to keep you focused on the task in hand during the call. You can consider asking any or all of the following questions:

♦ What treatment approach do you use?

♦ Are you able to provide . . . (your preferred type of therapy)?

♦ How much therapy experience do you have?

♦ How much experience in working with people with BPD do you have?

♦ Have you had any specialized training in treating people with BPD?

♦ What is your view of how therapy works?

♦ How long is therapy likely to last? (All the evidence-based psychotherapies have lasted at least one year and have been restricted to this time due to research constraints rather than clinical optimum, which would in most situations be longer than this.)

♦ Do you have other skills that may assist me?

♦ Are you happy to having an initial meeting—for both of us to assess whether we can work with each other?

♦ What are your fees?—or surcharge if applicable? (There is no point in causing yourself extra stress if you find the fee is beyond your abilities to pay.)

♦ Is the fee open to negotiation (if you cannot afford it)?

If you are comfortable with the answers to these questions, then make an appointment for a face-to-face meeting.

Preparing for the first face-to-face meeting with a potential therapist

Consider preparing for your first face-to-face meeting by writing down or highlighting the key points you want to know. Some of these points might be questions for yourself such as,

♦ Do I feel welcomed?

♦ Do I feel respected?

- Do I feel seen and heard?

- Do I feel safe?

- Do I feel comfortable?—Is this person easy to talk to?

- Does this person inspire my confidence?

- Does this person seem to know a way forward for me that makes sense to me?

Questions you might want answered from the therapist include:

- What is their philosophy about telephone calls between visits?

- How much time could I expect they will be away on vacation, study leave, etc?

- Would they allocate me a set weekly time?

- Fleshing out some of the questions asked briefly over the phone.

- Confirmation that they have their work supervised. (Supervision is a place where the therapist can discuss their work with a supervisor, to maximize their effectiveness. We would not recommend engaging in therapy with a therapist that does not have regular supervision.)

In preparing for the initial meeting, you can expect that both you and the therapist will be assessing whether you can work constructively together. To do this you will need to be prepared to share with the therapist information that will include

- Why you are seeking out therapy.

- What your aspirations and goals of therapy are.

- What your expectations of therapy are.

- Other information that the therapist will want to know.

If you are in therapy and considering changing therapist

If you are someone who is in a therapy relationship and considering changing your therapist, you will need to give serious attention to assessing the pros and cons of changing therapists. If your therapist has engaged in a major irretrievable violation of professional ethical codes of practice such as engaging in a sexual relationship with you, we encourage you to seek out a new therapist. When the situation is not so clear-cut, you will need to seek information that you can use to guide you wisely. Wherever possible, we encourage an approach where you explore with your therapist any concerns that you might have with a view to resolution and the therapy proceeding successfully.

When you raise concerns with your therapist, do not worry about your therapist feeling rejected. If they feel rejected, that is an issue for them to address themselves and in their supervision. You do not need to apologize for exploring your concerns. You have a right to assert yourself.

Having a therapist that works for you is very important. To achieve this goal may require a change of therapist but may also be better achieved by exploring the problem as you see it with your existing therapist. Most people with BPD have significant interpersonal relationship difficulties. It makes sense then that there may well be some interpersonal relationship difficulties with your therapist, especially in the earlier stages of treatment. If this is the case, both you and your therapist will need to work on your relationship so that treatment can proceed successfully. It will be really important that you do not make numerous shifts from one therapist to another when the solution lies in changes that you can make in the therapy relationship not the changing of the therapist. (*You can change your therapist but you still have to take yourself with you.*) Deciding to stay in your existing therapy relationship or changing to another therapist is a big decision that should be assessed and thoroughly explored.

 Comment from Wendy

I wasted many years by feeling powerless when looking for a therapist. I began work with the first person I contacted, without feeling I had any choice or power. If they were willing to see me I was just incredibly grateful. Likewise, I stayed in one untherapeutic therapy relationship too long because I believed the problems in the relationship were all mine. On the other hand, I have successfully stayed in a therapy relationship where interpersonal differences arose that we could talk about, demonstrating to me the value of 'talking it out'.

If I have one piece of advice: ***take charge of your recovery—do what is right for you***.

15

Developing a therapy agreement

 Key points

- It makes sense that you and your therapist explore and probably write down what the goals of therapy are.

- With an agreement, you know where you stand. An agreement can help you be clear about your role in your recovery and encourage you to be the author of your recovery.

- Successful therapy is about a genuine deeply collaborative relationship between two experts—expert professional and the person-in-recovery as expert about themselves.

You have now chosen a therapist and made a time to begin work with them. Well done! The next steps in the first few weeks of therapy are to clarify the therapy agreement and develop a relationship with your therapist.

Therapy goals

It makes good common sense that you and your therapist explore and probably write down what the goals of therapy are. This sounds obvious but often does not happen as both therapist and client attend to the strong emotions that are associated with a crisis, and another crisis, and yet another crisis, and 'forget' to get back to setting treatment goals. Setting treatment goals can guide both you and your therapist when therapy feels like you are in a ship in a storm at sea—it keeps the therapy ship on course. The storms need to be survived and the ship needs to stay as much as possible on course or get back on course as soon as possible after a storm. We also encourage goals to be named as specific behaviours that will be engaged in. In cognitive-behavioural therapies this will be standard but can also be applied well to other treatments. For example in a mentalization* treatment a behavioural goal will be for the client and therapist to target discussion where the client talks about thoughts, feelings, and behaviours with awareness and reflection.

Power, limits, boundaries, and being in charge of your recovery

You may, like many with BPD, have a history of having excessive inappropriate power exerted over you. If this is the case, it is understandable that you will be very sensitive around issues of power and determined that this power over the situation does not repeat itself.

You might be tempted to fight attempts on your therapist's part for clarity and structure around a treatment agreement, perceiving this as controlling; however, it is our experience that a treatment agreement can be one of the most useful processes in healing, by clarifying goals and expectations of both parties. With an agreement, you know where you stand, even if you dislike aspects of the agreement such as restrictions on telephone calls.

Instead of fearing power being used inappropriately against you, you might sometimes place too much power in the hands of others, thereby diminishing your own sense of authority. An agreement can help you be clear about your role in your recovery and encourage you to be the author of your recovery.

> **Explore how you can take charge of your recovery**

If you have a history of difficulty with your and others' limits/boundaries, an agreement also can provide clarity from the beginning of therapy that will mean that you are not always wondering where the limits are or what is OK and what is not OK.

Like many people with BPD, you may have a strong sense of justice and once you have given your word, unless compelling reasons exist, value sticking to your word. This strength can serve you well in reaping the benefits of therapy agreements.

Points to consider in establishing a therapy agreement

Points to consider in establishing a therapy agreement may include:

- Goals of therapy (short and long term), e.g. reduce distress, improve functioning, have children returned to your care, study, work, etc.

- When, where, and with what frequency sessions will be held.

- Expectations about cancellations (therapist and client). How much notice, consequences of missing sessions.

- Behaviours unacceptable during a session, e.g. violence, repeatedly intoxicated, telephone interruptions.

- Consequences of unacceptable behaviours.

- Contact outside session times—Is this available? If so during what hours and how often? What is the expected nature of contact, etc?

- Payment arrangements (pay at each session, monthly bill, etc.).

- Homework expectations, if applicable.

- Confirm confidentiality (you should be able to expect confidentiality from your therapist, with some exclusions as described in Chapter 12 ('What to expect from treatment').

- Procedures for vacations, alternative supports, crisis planning, hospitalization.

Therapy review

We value reviewing therapy every 3 or 6 months on a routine basis. The expectation here is that both therapist and person-in-recovery will have ideas about improvements that can be made to advance recovery. Having therapy review as routine shapes expectations, increasing the likelihood of therapist and person-in-recovery being open to possible changes.

Openness

A therapy agreement is to benefit you and your therapist, but especially you, so there is no point in 'cheating'—you will only be cheating yourself and possibly delaying your healing. It is important from the outset that you share any discomfort that you may have about the therapy agreement. You know yourself best, so it is in your interest to be honest about any patterns in past therapy of not acting in your own long-term best interest. Sharing these past patterns in an upfront manner enables you and your therapist to identify these patterns, not as something to be hidden at all cost, but as problems to be solved. It is much easier to solve a problem that is brought out into the light of day to be examined! As with many people with BPD, you may have a keen eye for loopholes in agreements, so be sure the wording in the agreement is very clear. Clearly stating behaviours that have been counter-productive for you in the past as problems to be solved will go some way to you taking charge of your recovery by closing loopholes that undermine your recovery.

Collaboration (working respectfully together towards common goals)

Successful therapy is about a genuine deeply collaborative relationship between two experts—expert professional and the person-in-recovery as expert about themselves. Successful therapy cannot happen with either party acting alone! You probably would not have entered therapy if you thought that you could have done it on your own and even the best therapist cannot do successful therapy without a client! Therapists, except in rare situations, are not the person-in-recovery's enemy.

16

Support network

 Key points

- Getting support from family and/or friends could be important for you and for your recovery; however, relationships may have become strained.

- Initially you may only have a few people in your support system. This is OK, as you can build your network as you go along.

- Family and friends can have a huge role in your recovery. They may be the people who know you best and may be the people who walk your journey most closely with you.

- It is important that you nurture and look after your support relationships.

- One way to help willing people in your support system is to help them understand the BPD condition.

- If you decide to inform support people of your treatment, it might be useful to let them know your treatment goals, and how they might be able to assist you in achieving these goals.

- Sharing along the way your gains and achievements, however small, will help those who support you feel valued for the effort they have put in to assist you.

- Build a reinforcing community that reinforces your skilful and effective behaviours.

Developing a support network

As one of the diagnostic criteria for BPD is having a pattern of intense and unstable relationships, you might have a weak support system around you. Getting support from family and/or friends is likely to be important for you and for your recovery; however, for some, relationships may have become strained.

It can be draining supporting someone with BPD. If you have too many eggs in one basket and are relying on one person for all your support, it is possible they may find the pressure too much, burn out and not want to see and support you, confirming your worst fears of rejection. Having support spread out across a broad-based network will be more likely to be effective for both you and your support people. On the other hand, you do not want to spread the support out too thinly, turning to just anyone and everyone. You will need to select a network that is likely to be reasonably and stably available to you, avoiding unstable 'fly by night' support relationships.

Who might be in your support network?

Those whom you might want in your support network include:

◆ family

◆ friends

◆ flatmates

◆ co-workers

◆ spiritual/religious advisors

◆ peer support workers

◆ GP

◆ therapist

◆ other mental health professionals

◆ crisis services

◆ teachers

◆ children's services.

Of course there are a huge variety of other people. Where possible, we encourage you to make use of relationships in your life, turning to therapists and mental health services only where this is not possible or is not effective. Initially you may only have a few people in your support system. This is OK, as you can build your network as you go along.

Role of family and friends in your support network

Where ongoing sexual, physical, or substantial verbal abuse is continuing, getting out of the abusive situation/s and relationships might be what is required in the first instance. On the other hand, family and friends can have a huge role in your recovery. They may be the people who know you best and may be the people who walk your journey most closely with you. When your doctor's office is closed and your therapist is on holiday, family and friends may be there for you. They may be the first people to notice subtle changes in your outlook (early warning signs), sometimes even before you. They may be able successfully to cheer you on at times.

Family and friends are those most likely to bear the brunt of your anger and frustration. They may be the ones on the receiving end of your black and white, all or nothing thinking—being seen by you as angels one moment and enemy the next. Hopefully they will also be the subject of your affection and share the fun times along the way.

It may be that some of you are estranged from families who have done the best that they knew how and distanced themselves from you or you from them. While there are no guarantees, relationships can be mended and as you begin to heal and your emotions become more regulated, family and friends might respond positively when contact is resumed.

> Relationships can be repaired, and the fact that you are making steps toward changing your life is more likely to gain approval from those around you

 Comment from Wendy

Unfortunately for many years of my recovery, I was estranged from my family and friends through my most difficult times. Eventually I was able to repair some of these relationships and this in turn assisted my recovery further.

Looking after your support network

Supporting and rewarding your support people

It must be remembered that the journey is a difficult one for our support people too—like us, they also benefit, as we all do, from nurturing and encouragement. It is important that we look after these relationships. Doing small (or large) things for family and/or friends when we are not in crisis will communicate to them that we value them.

There is often no better reward than simply, 'Thank you—I have had a better day because of what you have done for me'. Saying a simple 'thank you' takes just a moment, is achievable, requiring only a small amount of energy, and will in most cases be well received as the person identifies that we care about them and have them and their efforts in mind. Another small example is complimenting the person on what they are wearing or what they have done that day.

If you don't feel able to verbalize these feelings, a small card in the mail does wonders and will bring a smile to almost anyone's face. A card or small gift indicates to the other person that you have been mindful of them by your personal investment of time and energy.

If we get into a row and have behaved in a manner that we regret, we need to see if we can repair the relationship. A simple apology can go a long way to softening people's hearts. However, there are usually limits to how many apologies a person will be able to accept without us changing our behaviours. Sometimes we might want to consider an overcorrection. This is where we not only make up for behaviours we regret (correction) but go further and make the situation even better for the person we have upset than before we engaged in the behaviour that we regret. For example, if we use a friend's car without permission, we can correct it by returning the car and making an apology. Overcorrection might involve also cleaning, washing, and polishing the car.

Finally, sharing along the way our gains and achievements, however small, will help those who support us feel valued for the effort they have put in to assist us. We can help them feel that their efforts have been worthwhile by sharing our successes and how much we have appreciated their assistance.

If we can help our support people feel valued, in addition to bringing pleasure to them, they are also more likely to continue supporting us. Good for them, good for us.

Long haul, boundaries, and limits

BPD is not a short-term condition with a quick fix. Just as you and your therapist are in it for the long haul, it is important that *you* support *your* support network to also be in it for the long haul.

Knowing what is and what is not OK for each individual support person will help both you and your support people set healthy limits/boundaries that you can all live with, decreasing the likelihood of either or both parties burning out. Sticking within these agreed upon limits is likely to increase the chances of gaining their respect and yours. Once you have helped your support people last the distance then you all can share in the joys of your recovery.

'I' statements, and healthy non-judgemental assertion

'I' statements tend to be less offensive, generate more understanding, and ultimately be more effective when speaking to a person who you feel has hurt or wronged you. 'I felt hurt when you . . .' rather than 'You hurt me!' What we are looking for here is a non-judgemental description of events and avoiding assuming that we can know other people's thoughts, emotions, and motivations without them telling us. This sounds simple but is not necessarily easy to do, and will require practice.

Understanding the BPD condition

One way to help willing people in your support system is to help them understand the BPD condition. Giving them a book such as this (although this is designed for you, the person with BPD) or other material on BPD may enable them to understand you and your inner turmoil better, which could then lead to better support for you when the going gets tough. One woman who has recovered from BPD writes how her mother was able to be more effective in helping her when she better understood the BPD condition:

 Comment from Wendy

I might have said that I feel really ugly and did not want to leave the house and previously my mother would have said that was exactly the reason that I should go out—face my fears. While this had been true, because it was done on its own without also validating my experience, I had not been able to benefit from her well-meaning advice. Once my mother knew more about BPD, she was better able to step back and validate me by saying something like, 'That must be terrible, feeling that way. Is there anything that I can do to help?' Having them understand really opened up the communication between me and my family. They felt like they were helping me—and they were!

Printed with permission of Alison (pseudonym)

Involvement in your treatment

You will need to consider the advantages and disadvantages of having those supporting you informed about your treatment and/or involved in treatment planning and/or meeting your therapist. For some, a bit of distance between your therapy and your support people is what you require, maintaining the privacy of your therapy. For others, having support people involved can lead to all parties understanding and valuing each other better, and support people understanding your treatment better and how they can best assist you.

If you decide to inform support people of your treatment, it might be useful to let them know your treatment goals, and how they might be able to assist you in achieving these goals. Ask them if there is anything they need clarification about or feel uneasy about. Developing a Wellness Action Recovery Plan (http://www.copelandcenter.com was a suitable website when this book was written in 2007), which clearly tells your support people what you might want from them under various circumstances, can be a useful strategy.

Whether or not you involve support people in treatment planning, having a written note that provides those supporting you with some ideas of things they can say or suggest that you would find helpful when the going gets tough might help them feel a little more in control and help them offer support that is actually useful to you. Having issues out in the open before there is a crisis can be productive, supporting your support people to be there for the long haul.

Building a reinforcing community

We all like getting rewards or reinforcement when we do things well. You can help yourself by asking others in your community to reward or reinforce you (perhaps, for example, with words of encouragement or time together) when you have been skilful and effective in doing things that advance your treatment goals and not to reinforce or reward you when you are doing things that are ineffective or unskilful. You and your community will need to agree ahead of time what behaviours will be reinforced and what behaviours will not be reinforced.

17

Assessment

⮕ Key points

◆ While the assessment and planning stages can feel like you are not getting 'treatment', they are essential foundations for successful treatment and can be some of the most important sessions you might have.

◆ A skilled therapist will be mindful of taking things at a pace that best suits you.

◆ One of the most important areas of the assessment phase is for your therapist to clearly understand your strengths, problems, and therapy goals clearly.

◆ Openness is the best policy—this information is to help both of you plan for treatment.

General information

When you first start seeing a therapist, they and you will begin the process of getting to know you through a thorough assessment. You can expect this phase, which usually takes more than one session, to be a mixture of connecting with each other, and your therapist gathering and you sharing factual information about yourself.

Foundation of treatment

Treatment can be conceptually layered, with each layer having its foundations in the layer below:

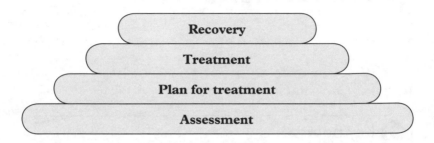

While the assessment and planning stages can feel like you are not getting 'treatment', they are essential foundations for successful treatment and can sometimes be the most important treatment sessions you might have. Have patience—it is for your benefit in the long run.

Surviving crises and still completing assessment

It might be difficult for you and your therapist to complete the assessment due to pressing urgent constant crises taking your attention. Crises, of course, need to be survived and somehow got through. Also, do try to set up some time where you can discuss things without a current crisis so that the assessment can be completed. Unexpected and unwanted surprises await both you and your therapist if you both lurch from one crisis to another without an adequate assessment ever taking place.

Pace and trust

The assessment can be a difficult time as information covered might lead to distress. With this in mind, it is important for you to be mindful of your feelings and for both you and your therapist to pace the information sharing and gathering.

The assessment phase can be difficult for those who struggle with issues of trust. You might feel like you are baring your soul, so it makes sense that you will be a little wary. You are sharing who you are with someone you have only recently met, yet it is incredibly important that they do get to know you.

Others who trust too readily might be tempted to share too much too quickly.

A skilled therapist will be mindful of taking things at a pace that best suits you and might be willing to leave areas that you find difficult until later in the assessment, allowing trust to build as you get to know each other. Reflect on how much sharing will be optimal for you in these first sessions. If you feel it is all moving too fast, and you are becoming overwhelmed, you need to say so—take charge.

Information sharing and gathering during assessment

Goals

One of the most important areas of the assessment phase is for your therapist to understand your problems and your therapy goals clearly. What do you want to achieve from therapy? The two of you will then need to explore whether your goals and your therapist's goals are in agreement or what common goals the two of you can agree to work on. Discussing these goals will guide the two of you in developing your plan for treatment.

 Comment from Wendy

I found it difficult to know what I wanted from life except for 'I want to feel better'. It was too painful for me to consider and entertain dreams, hopes, and what I wanted in my life as my experience had been that most goals I had previously set had led to failure. Eventually I got around this by setting small and achievable goals with my clinicians, and once we had worked on these and I had developed a glimmer of confidence that I could achieve goals, we were able to set bigger and more meaningful goals. It is OK to start out small.

Skills and strengths

Your therapist will probably want to know your psychological skills, behaviours you are good at, other strengths, and aspects of yourself that make you hardy and flexible (resilient) as a base from which you can grow and develop the skills you have yet to develop. If you have difficulty acknowledging your self-worth it may be useful to have a friend assist you as they may be more objective about your strengths. Your therapist will also probably want to know what energizes you and what you enjoy as a base to grow and develop the things you do not yet enjoy or are not yet energized by. Discussing your skills will guide the two of you in developing your plan for treatment.

Function

Your therapist will want to know how you function on a day to day basis and what your 'average' day is like. Many of us find that we can function well on some days and less well on other days. Your therapist will want to know your roles (work, parent, daughter, son, friend, caregiver etc.), and how well you function in each of these roles. Many of us find we can function really well in one role and less well in another (e.g. function well at work and less well at home, or vice versa). Discussing your level of function will guide the two of you in developing your plan for treatment.

Current and past treatment

Your therapist will want information about any other mental health care you are currently receiving or have received in the past. Information as to what was helpful and unhelpful will help the two of you learn from your past therapy and mental health treatment experiences and plan accordingly so that the therapy you are engaging in can be as productive as possible. Information from current and past treatments will guide the two of you in developing your plan for treatment.

Relationships

As many people with BPD struggle with relationships, your therapist will want information about your relationships and any notable relationship patterns that you are aware of. Your therapist will want to know what social supports you currently have; formal, informal, professional, and casual, and how these are helpful to you or not. Information from relationship patterns, including those with past therapists, will guide the two of you in developing your plan for treatment.

Personality style

Your therapist will want an understanding of how you make your way in the world—your personality style. For example, where do you sit on the continuum from reserved to extroverted, impulsive to rigidly organized, bottling up anger to lashing out, and from excessive leaning on others to excessive self-reliance? Remember, openness is the best policy—this information is to help both of you plan for treatment.

Behaviours

Your therapist will want to know, where applicable, about suicide attempts, self-harm, alcohol, drug, gambling, and eating problems. Information of great use to both of you will be understanding past patterns, so that both of you can explore skilful solutions that you might use when you pick up early warning signs. Again, openness is the best policy—this information is to help both of you plan for treatment.

18

Treatment goals and treatment plan

→ Key points

- Because BPD affects every individual in a different way, everyone's goals arc different.

- We encourage goals to be broken down into and named as specific behaviours that will be engaged in.

- None of us has a life that is filled with only happy moments—this is not a realistic goal. What is realistic is to be able to get to a place where we look forward with anticipation to enough future events or where we go to bed at night with a sense of 'today was OK', 'better than OK', and occasionally 'wonderful'.

- Your treatment plan is an agreed upon plan for recovery that clarifies both your treatment goals and treatment pathways, and steps towards achieving these goals.

Treatment goals

Because BPD affects every individual in a different way, everyone's goals are different.

You may have entered treatment because you want life to be more pleasurable. Steps along the way will need to include finding ways of surviving your current distress and developing new skills for putting in place behaviours that are likely to generate more pleasure in the short and long term. In the short term this may be engaging in your favourite pleasurable activities and in the long term improving relationships and work-related activities.

Your goal of treatment may be to have a life that is more meaningful and purposeful. Steps along the way will need to include knowing what you want from life and planning activities to increase the chances of engaging in meaningful and/or purposeful activities.

Your treatment goals may be to learn new skills to manage your emotions better so that you can feel in control of your emotions rather than them being in control of you. Steps along the way will include learning to identify emotions, accept emotions, and engage in activities that generate more pleasing emotions.

You may have entered treatment after having your children removed from your care, and therefore your goal may be to get your children back. To achieve this final goal you will be needing to meet goals along the way, such as feeling stable enough to get out of bed each morning and then to run a household.

You may have had a major fall out with family members, or a partner, and your goal may be to learn to develop and maintain healthy relationships with others. To do this you will need to meet goals along the way such as regulating your emotions, taming impulsivity, and learning the interpersonal skills required for maintaining healthy relationships.

Marsha Linehan (1993b), who developed DBT, describes a number of skills to learn on your journey through treatment. These skills include distress tolerance (learning to cope with and manage difficult times without making things worse), interpersonal effectiveness (learning to develop and maintain healthy relationships), and emotion regulation (learning to be in control of your emotions).

As we have stated earlier, we encourage goals to be broken down into and named as specific behaviours that will be engaged in. Examples include telephoning friends as the behaviour that will lead to improved relationships, or recording or discussing thoughts, feelings, and behaviours that will lead to increased awareness and problem-solving skills.

None of us has a life that is filled with only happy moments—this is not a realistic goal. What is realistic is to be able to get to a place where we look forward with anticipation to enough future events or where we go to bed at night with a sense of 'today was OK', 'better than OK', and occasionally 'wonderful'. Your goal may be to move from a life that is only just bearable to one that becomes more easily bearable, to one that is filled with enough pleasure and meaning. Whatever your individual goals that motivated you to seek help or pick up this book, it is likely that you are motivated to leave therapy or treatment with the achievable goal of having, what DBT has as a core treatment goal; 'a life worth living'.

> **A satisfying life is achievable!**

Treatment plan

What is your treatment plan?

Your treatment plan is an agreed upon plan for your recovery that clearly states both your treatment goals and treatment pathways, and steps towards achieving these goals.

Collaborative

A treatment plan is developed in a collaborative manner by you and your therapist or you and the clinicians involved in your treatment and recovery. (This means you each have meaningful input into the plan. It might be that family and friends are involved in some way that clarifies their role in your recovery and your role in supporting them to support you.)

To document or not?

If you are involved with several clinicians perhaps in a public mental health service, documenting your treatment plan can assist those involved in your treatment to be well informed. This document might be held on your file with a copy for yourself. Many insurance companies require documented treatment plans.

Multi-treating agency

In a multi-treating agency, you will want your documented treatment plan to state the roles of each person in your treatment, how and when you contact them, and what you can expect from them and what they can expect from you. Some examples of the types of people in your treatment team may be your therapist, prescribing doctor, family doctor, 'case manager' (sic), crisis clinicians, inpatient clinicians, and possibly others such as social service or children's service workers.

Boundaries/limits, contingencies (what happens after), crisis information, and review in a multi-treating agency

You will want your treatment plan to inform clinicians of agreed upon boundaries/limits put in place to enhance your outcome such as what happens after self-harm or arriving at therapy intoxicated. You will want your treatment plan to inform clinicians of things you are likely to find helpful and unhelpful at times of crisis, if applicable. You will want your plan to state when it will be reviewed, and how review will measure progress, especially against your and your therapist's agreed upon goals.

 Comment from Wendy

It was a significant turning point in my recovery when a group of concerned and insightful mental health professionals in various teams in a public mental health service began to meet and discuss how they could best deliver their services to develop my own coping skills while still leaving me feeling supported. At first I was sure these meetings were a conspiracy and, when first presented with my treatment plan, was dubious to say the least. Having a treatment plan completely changed the focus—no longer were others responsible for my life and safety. Instead I was responsible for my own feelings and subsequent actions.

I had clear expectations of where my treatment was heading and consequences for some of my more destructive behaviours, and the team had clear guidelines, providing a path for us all to share and follow. Prolonged admissions under compulsion were suddenly a part of my past and, while terrified, I responded positively to the control I was now being handed. Slowly I got over the sense of conspiracy, feeling part of that team, and considered my views and opinions were listened to and heard. I would not have recovered without this plan for treatment.

19

Therapy relationship

➲ Key points

◆ A good therapeutic relationship will be one of the keys to your recovery.

◆ Treat the relationship with basic respect and honesty, be assertive, keep to your agreements and your therapist's limits.

◆ Ride impulsive urges to fire your therapist except in extraordinary circumstances.

◆ Trust will hopefully develop, and you will be on the road to your recovery.

A 'therapeutic relationship' is one you have with any of the clinicians you work with and is probably of greatest relevance with your therapist.

Differences from other relationships

It is part of the nature of the therapy relationship that your therapist will know more about you than you will about them to enable both of you to focus primarily on you and your needs. While the therapist has important rights, the relationship is set up primarily for your benefit. The relationship is dedicated to understanding you and assisting you make the necessary changes required to meet agreed upon goals.

It is a place set up to assist your feeling safe in discussing your struggles and a place where you can safely learn and practise new skills. The relationship has boundaries and limits that are as open, clear, and overt as is possible. Not all eventualities can be pre-planned for, so some boundaries and limits will need to be discussed as events unfold.

The relationship is different from other relationships in that it is openly an important part of your and the therapist's job to work on interpersonal issues in your relationship where relevant. It is a relationship that will not necessarily be easy for you or for your therapist as you might be entering the relationship with a limited range of effective interpersonal skills that are likely to manifest in the therapy relationship. Provided these difficulties are not extreme, such as physical assault or continuous verbal abuse, the therapist and you will have agreed to work through these difficulties. This 'working' on the relationship will involve practising improving interpersonal skills so that the relationship moves to becoming increasingly effective.

Like any relationship, it takes time to develop, and needs to be nurtured, reflected upon, and have attention paid to it.

Getting to know one another

As a therapeutic relationship is likely to be started with an appointment; it has a somewhat artificial start, compared with other relationships in your life. You may know a little about your therapist (qualifications, fees, areas of expertise) and they may know a little about you (referral) before the two of you meet.

The first few weeks of therapy will be spent getting to know each other. As discussed in Chapter 17, your therapist will need lots of information about you, in order to help you, and you will need to get to know the therapist and develop some level of trust. Beware of the danger of trusting excessively and too quickly, as this can lead to reluctance to attend further sessions if you feel too open and vulnerable.

During the first few weeks, the two of you will discuss treatment goals, expectations, availability, limits of availability, and limits of the relationship, culminating in a plan for treatment that may or may not be documented.

Making the most of your therapy relationship

Like any relationship, the therapeutic relationship takes a combination of respect, honesty, and trust to work. There are some things you can do to maximize the relationship working best for you.

Respect

Respect is a two-way process. Respect has different depths. Minimal respect is what you can expect from any professional; however, deep respect is what you need to aim for, as this will most likely have a powerful healing effect for you.

We are not talking here of deep respect because of accomplishments but rather deep respect because you are a courageous human being who, despite emotional pain, is willing to engage with another human being in a shared journey of discovery and change.

> **You are courageous**

The very fact that you are dealing with raw or turbulent emotions means that you are likely to have strong feelings and to express your strong feelings. Assuming it is warranted, show your therapist respect by your behaviours. *Never* resort to violence—to yourself, the room around you, or towards your therapist. If you feel like lashing out in a physical or verbally abusive manner, try to discuss the issue and gain assistance to deal with the feelings in a manner that is safe and respectful for both you and your therapist.

Another means of showing basic respect for your therapist and the relationship is to show up on time, and give plenty of notice if you need to cancel. You and your therapist might have agreed that you attend sessions, except in an extreme emergency, in a clear mind free from intoxicants (alcohol, drugs). The therapeutic relationship is to benefit you, so you need to take responsibility for these things. Not to do so will undermine your own healing.

Openness

Openness in this context refers to not telling half-truths, providing part information, looking for technical loopholes in agreements, and deliberately telling significant lies, which of course will be harmful to any relationship.

Deep collaboration (working together) is genuinely respectful—half answers deprive both of you from working collaboratively together. Be as open as you are safely able to be with your therapist. Your therapist can only work with the information you share, and giving half answers, providing part information, and looking for technical loopholes is unlikely to generate the trust and respect that you want from your therapist.

Are you committed to deep collaboration? If so, you will need to be honest and open.

Boundaries and limits

The best time to express your dislike of specific boundaries and limits is at the time of establishing your therapy agreements. Once you and your therapist have discussed and agreed upon the boundaries and limits around your relationship, stick to them or, if unhappy with them, discuss them with your therapist before breaking the agreement.

One way for therapists to care about you and your relationship is by ensuring that they don't burn out. A burnt-out clinician will be de-energized, unenthusiastic, have difficulty retaining necessary hopefulness when things get tough, and be significantly restricted in their ability to help you heal.

> **You do not want your clinicians to burn out**

You and your therapist will have agreed upon actions for you to take if emergencies occur outside of the agreed upon contact times. Your agreement might or might not include contacting your therapist during agreed upon hours if you need to repair your relationship, for skills coaching, or are in crisis. If calls outside of sessions are part of your agreement, save them for what you have agreed to—unnecessary overuse can overload your therapist. If your agreement is that you are able to call outside of therapy sessions until 5pm, don't be tempted to put it off until three minutes to five, just to see if your therapist really cares.

It is their job to make sure that they remain energized and enthusiastic (not burnt out) by staying within boundaries and limits that they can sustain over the long haul. It is also your job to make sure they don't burn out by your staying within agreed upon boundaries and limits. Too much pushing and you might succeed in pushing them away—the thing you want the very least. Being in the driver's seat and taking control of your treatment means sticking to the agreements that have been made at least until such time as you have been able to re-negotiate.

On the other hand, insufficient use of crisis calls can also be a problem, preventing you from getting appropriate assistance.

> **Explore how you can take charge of your recovery**

Asserting yourself

Stating your feelings and talking them through to some degree of resolution is an important process in your healing. If you feel hurt or not understood by your therapist, assert yourself and respectfully discuss this with them. Your therapist is a human being not a magician—the only things they will know for sure about you are what you tell them.

> ## Do not assume your therapist can read your mind!

Believing that they 'should' be able to read your mind or pick up on your body or facial cues leaves you open to being misunderstood. It is your responsibility to question them if you do not understand what was meant, or to clarify if you think you have been misunderstood. This is an important relationship in your healing—we encourage you to raise assertively with your therapist concerns you may have about the relationship. This can be a positive experience, serving as both practice and a model for relationships outside therapy.

Resisting the urge to fire your therapist impulsively—commitment

We encourage you to make a commitment to yourself that you are on this journey of recovery for the long haul, and that if you feel like leaving therapy you will do it in a planned way, in collaboration with your therapist. Many people with BPD drop out of therapy prematurely, when feeling misunderstood or rejected. Recognizing and acknowledging feeling rejected to oneself can result in productive discussion and repair with your therapist. Because feeling rejected is so painful it is understandable that recognizing and acknowledging this feeling will be painful; however, leaving therapy without discussing the issues will not advance your healing. Unfortunately, you, the person-in-recovery, are the person who gets hurt in this situation. This is not to say that you should never leave a therapist unilaterally, rather that any such plans are considered and thorough except in extraordinary circumstances, such as where your therapist is in obvious flagrant breach of ethical codes of practice such as having sex with you.

> ## Resist the urge to fire your therapist impulsively for long enough to reflect

Comment from Wendy

I believe a very large part of where I am today is due to two therapeutic relationships I had. Sometimes the two people were fantastic—they were there when I needed them and I didn't have to put on my 'coping face' for them—sometimes they were not all I wanted and they were not available when I wanted them. But, they kept their commitments, doing what they said they would and they stuck with me right through my journey till I built a satisfying life.

20

Taking charge of your recovery

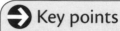 **Key points**

- Taking charge of your role in your therapy might sound scary; however, it will have a major impact on your recovery. When you achieve small steps towards your recovery, you can enjoy the credit for making this happen. Small tasks achieved will have been created by *you* and will be able to be claimed by *you*.

- Now is the best time to take charge of whatever you can to make the changes necessary to create the circumstances to make your life different.

- Discuss and clarify with your therapist what you can do, what they can do, what you can expect from them, and what they can expect from you.

- Choosing to take charge of your therapy will be a cornerstone of your healing and you will be on the way towards recovery.

Your therapist is bound by their profession to provide therapy at a reasonable standard, supporting you in your endeavours to reflect, understand yourself, and learn and practise new behaviours and ways of being. You on the other hand are not bound by any code of behaviour, except that of your own values (and society's laws). Taking charge of your role in your therapy might sound scary; however, it will have a major impact on your recovery. When you achieve small steps towards your recovery, you can enjoy the credit for making this happen. Small tasks achieved will have been created by *you* and will be able to be claimed by *you*. You will build up your view of yourself as a competent human being.

You may very well not have had the power previously, say as a child, to have made your life different. Now is the best time to take charge of whatever you can to make the changes necessary to create the circumstances to make your life different.

It will be worth discussing and clarifying with your therapist what you can do, what they can do, what you can expect from them and what they can expect from you. Finding the balance between what you and your therapist are responsible for is like balancing a see-saw (teeter-totter) with ever changing weights. Having these issues as part of your treatment plan can guide you and your therapist to behaviours that are likely to advance your recovery.

While it is appropriate that your therapist engages in behaviours to help you with your distress, it is important that their behaviours encourage you to learn new skills as well as surviving current crises. As much as possible, your therapist will want to support you in your endeavours, and not get in the way of your learning, by doing things for you that you can do for yourself. Occasionally your therapist might need to do something for you where the stakes are very high and your skills are low. Getting this balance right will be challenging and will need to be talked about if your and your therapist's views differ.

Linehan, who developed DBT, uses the metaphor of life resembling being dealt a series of cards (Linehan, 1993b). It is great fun to play our cards when we are dealt a set of cards that we like and much harder when we are dealt a lousy set of cards. The task is not to throw our cards in when we get dealt a set of cards different from what we would like. The task is to play each set of cards we are dealt as best we can and wait to see what the next set of cards brings.

 Comment from Wendy

. . . it occurred to me, maybe for the first time, that he was not responsible for my recovery: as a psychologist his job was not to make me better but rather to act as an advocate between me and my condition, to equip me with the tools necessary to make myself better. He could provide me with the knowledge and insight to understand and eventually manage my

> condition, but he could not do the hard work for me. It was up to me to take his advice. It was up to me to do the things to ensure that I stayed well. This battle was mine and mine alone. I was in the driving seat, controlling the action; my therapist and all the assorted medical professionals involved with me were mere passengers that had come along for the ride.
>
> Desmond (2004)

You may have had a variety of emotions and reactions reading through this book. When you started reading the book you may have excitedly thought, 'Help is here at last, someone will understand, make sense of my world for me and fix my problems'. Later you may have thought, 'I am not better yet so this book must be useless'. We encourage you to find those parts of the book that will be helpful, adding them to your repertoire of resources.

 Comment from Wendy

My situation was, in my mind, desperate and without hope. I really wanted someone or something to cure me and did not realize till much later that the answer lay within myself. If there was some way to have discovered this earlier, I would have saved myself a lot of trouble and distress and shortened my time to recovery.

Explore how you can take charge of your recovery

21

Power struggles and beyond

> ## ➔ Key points
>
> ◆ Both you and your therapist have responsibilities to contribute towards collaboration, thereby reducing the risk of power struggles.
>
> ◆ When two people have differing views about important matters, it is inevitable that conflict will arise.
>
> ◆ By expecting and discussing difference you can move through and *beyond power struggles* to a successful effective therapy.

A snag that may occur in attempting to take charge of your recovery are power struggles between you and those trying to help you. When two people have differing views, a conviction and commitment to deep collaboration (working together towards agreed goals) will help move through the power struggles to life beyond power struggles.

People with BPD, like anyone else, have pride; however, in fighting for control we can back ourselves into a corner, sometimes with very poor outcomes. If we feel that others are trying to control us, it makes sense that we will try to avoid being controlled. A temptation exists to do this in a manner that 'cuts off our nose to spite our face' or in a manner of 'shooting ourselves in the foot'. That is, we end up with control that is counter-productive or even devastating. For example, because it is extremely difficult for others to control what you do to your body, you might self-harm as a way of staying in control. Another example is to tell people that you are suicidal and then to refuse offers of assistance. This can sometimes lead to an escalation of extremely dangerous behaviour. ***This is a lose–lose situation***. If this applies to you, it is essential and reasonably urgent that you find other less dangerous ways of feeling and being in control.

Both you and your therapist have responsibilities to contribute towards collaboration (working together towards agreed goals), thereby reducing the risk of power struggles. Collaborative clarifying and agreeing on areas of responsibility at times of calm will increase the likelihood of an expected response at times of crisis. Having an expected response is likely to increase our sense of being in control. We are not suggesting that collaboration is an easy task. When two people have differing views about important matters, it is inevitable that conflict will arise. The challenge is to engage overtly, assertively, and respectfully with the person you are in conflict with, seeking out a solution that both parties can live with. For therapy to be successful, you will need your therapist, and your therapist will need you. If either of you drop out, therapy cannot be successful! By expecting and discussing differences you can move through and *beyond power struggles* to a successful effective therapy.

 Comment from Wendy

It still saddens me that I wasted several futile years embroiled in power struggles with clinicians. While I desperately wanted clinicians to fix my problems, I also simultaneously was petrified to acknowledge any reasonable (or unreasonable) authority of their professional knowledge and experience. At times, struggling to solve this dilemma, I would strive to be totally and solely in charge of the relationship with my clinicians. One way I would do this was to communicate intense distress and then refuse offers of assistance. On occasions this led to involuntary treatment. I would then indignantly blame them for my loss of freedom and would fight against them all the way. I desperately wanted them to take control and responsibility for my life—only to be angered when they tried to help. I wasted precious time and energy by concealing my needs and not being willing to work collaboratively alongside clinicians, rather than fight them for power.

22

Prioritizing your therapy focus

➜ Key points

♦ When you first enter therapy, you and your therapist will most probably focus on getting to know one another, clarifying treatment goals and developing a plan for treatment.

♦ Your safety and the safety of others, if relevant, will be of paramount importance, as will be the relationship with your therapist.

♦ Once safety has been achieved, the next focus will be improving the quality of your life.

♦ In therapy sessions, you will be encouraged to be yourself and reflect upon your internal world and your relationships with those external to you.

♦ Sometimes BPD can take over your life. If this is the case, you will need to take your life back, piece by piece. While you might need to pace yourself during your therapy, it is important also that you hang on as much as possible to your productive life outside of therapy.

♦ Finally, it will be time to take all that you have learned about yourself, relationships, and the world, and move on.

Stages of therapy

Of course, like most things in life, healing does not happen in a straight line nor overnight, and you are likely to move between different stages of recovery at various times. This is not a race, so do not be tempted to set yourself up to fail with excessively high expectations.

When you first enter therapy, you and your therapist will most probably focus on getting to know one another, clarifying treatment goals, and developing a plan for treatment. You will then focus attention on exploring how you can achieve your goals. This can feel overwhelming, thinking 'where do we start?'

Safety

Your safety and the safety of others, if relevant, will be of paramount importance, as will be the relationship with your therapist. Therapy is likely to focus on assisting you stabilize your emotional state and learn new skills to deal with strong feelings and keeping yourself safe. Therapy will involve you and your therapist finding solutions to agreed upon treatment goals that include healthier alternative ways to deal with your strong feelings. In some therapies your relationship with your therapist will be a core means of achieving this stability. Cognitive-behavioural therapies, such as DBT, will have you doing 'homework' and filling out a diary card that monitors problems of safety such as suicidal thoughts, self-harm, substance use, assault, and urges to these behaviours if applicable to you. Therapy will explore solutions for these problems. If you are in standard DBT, in addition to individual therapy, you will also attend a skills group that teaches skills of living, including dealing with strong emotions. Preparing for crises is another way for you to work on how to keep yourself safe and maximize stability (see 'Preparing for crises' in Chapter 23).

Quality of life

Once safety has been achieved, the next focus will be improving the quality of your life. Therapy will now target decreasing behaviours that are a problem such as gambling, binge eating, and social anxiety, or increasing behaviours such as those that embrace independence, dignity, and meaningful activity. In all therapies you will be encouraged to generalize into your wider community any changes that you make in the therapy sessions.

In therapy sessions, you will be encouraged to be yourself and reflect upon your internal world and your relationships with those external to you. Being yourself may include being sad, happy, anxious, angry, content, and other emotions. Reflecting upon your internal world will include reflections on these different emotional states, what prompted them and what you might do as a result of these emotional states. You will reflect on the chain of events (cues/triggers, thoughts, emotions, behaviours) that lead to problems seeking out alternative solutions.

You will be encouraged to express your feelings about your therapist as a core part of some treatments and, if you are in a cognitive-behavioural therapy, as a means of addressing any problems that might arise in the therapy relationship.

Trauma work

Once you have reasonable stability in your life and feel reasonably in control of your emotions, you might want to move on to exploring past trauma as a means of further addressing current difficulties. Once you have learned to keep yourself safe, and developed stability and skills to deal with strong feelings, you will be more equipped to deal with the strong and often distressing emotions that trauma work may activate/set off. Trauma work takes place in the second stage of DBT and in most other therapies once stabilization has been achieved.

Eye movement desensitization and reprocessing (EMDR) has been shown to be effective in treating ongoing negative effects of trauma. EMDR therapists deliberately have the client engaging in rapid eye movements while recalling memories of past trauma, believing that the eye movements are a critical part of the positive effect. On the other hand, it is the opinion of many others that this is not due to any specific effects of eye movements *per se* but due to the effects of exposing oneself to memories of the traumatic material and having anxiety lessen with time that is the critical part of achieving the positive effect. This deliberate exposure to trauma memories while ensuring that anxiety decreases is at the core of behavioural and trauma therapies.

Many people with BPD have a history of physical, sexual, or emotional abuse or trauma. The question is often asked, 'If the abuse or trauma I suffered caused me to be like this, surely I can just talk about the abuse/trauma, get over it, and all will be well'. We wish this were the case. Dealing with past abuse or trauma can be a challenging process, bringing up strong distressing emotions. If you are significantly distressed when starting therapy, and the only therapy you do is intense talking about past trauma, it is likely that you will not have the skills to cope with strong intense emotions generated and possible impulsive urges. For this reason, we believe that specifically and intensively talking about the details of past trauma is best done when you have developed a trusting relationship with your therapist, learned ways to tame your impulsivity, and developed an array of skills to tolerate distress and manage turbulent emotions. This is not to say that your trauma and the importance of the trauma should not be respectfully acknowledged, rather that timing when to talk about this is critical.

Some people with histories of trauma make robust (strong) recoveries choosing to not focus specifically on trauma work, while others choose to engage in trauma work later in therapy to deepen and strengthen their recovery.

Pacing

Consider the following story:

> A lecturer teaching stress management to his students gets them to raise a glass of water and asks 'How heavy do you think this glass of water is?' The students' answers range from 100 g to 1000 g. He asks them to continue holding the glass for a minute asking the same question, and then for five, ten and twenty minutes asking the same question each time. The glass of water does not change in actual scientific weight, however, as the students increasingly agitatedly declare, it *feels* heavier and heavier. The absolute weight matters less to the students than the perception of the weight.

The perception of the weight depends on how long we hold it. If we hold it for a minute it is OK. If we hold it for an hour, we will have very sore arms. If we hold it for a day, we will be in agony—and our arms are likely to need treatment. The weight does not change, but the longer we hold it the heavier it becomes.

In life we carry our burdens and if we don't put them down some of the time, the burden becomes increasingly heavy. What we have to do is take responsibility for pacing ourselves, putting down our burdens and resting for a while from time to time before picking up again. In putting the burden down, we can get on with some of the ordinary things in our lives—work, reading a child a story, or taking a walk. The load can then be picked up again when we are rested.

When we put the load down, we remain in charge and responsible, keeping an eye on it, ready to pick it up if necessary earlier than planned. In taking charge of pacing ourselves periodically, we can refresh ourselves, re-charge our batteries, and be better able to carry on.

Getting on with life outside therapy

Sometimes BPD can take over your life. If this is the case, you will need to take your life back, and create your non-BPD life piece by piece. While you might need to pace yourself during your therapy, it is important also that you hang on as much as possible to your productive life outside of therapy.

During your therapy journey, you will need to develop and maintain a life outside of therapy that is satisfying. This may include relationships, interests/hobbies, study, or work-related activities. We encourage you to get on with life outside of therapy as much as you are able throughout the different stages of your therapy. Getting on with life might be specifically targeted in therapy, looking for specific solutions, or it might happen as a natural generalization (broadening) of other changes you are making in therapy.

Leaving therapy

It is quite likely that the amount of therapy you can access will be restricted by your finances, insurance company, or public mental health service. In these situations, you will need to explore with your therapist how you can make the most of what *is* available to you.

For those who do not have these restrictions, the time to leave therapy is when therapy is impeding other aspects of what has become a healthy life. That is, attending therapy costs too much money and takes too much time and gets in the way of other more important matters in your life. Ideally you and your therapist will come to the conclusion together about the right time to leave therapy. Leaving therapy needs to be carefully considered, well discussed with your therapist, and be planned for a time in the future that allows for a substantial period to talk about and come to terms with your probably strong and mixed feelings about leaving. It is quite likely that you will feel some anxiety, some sadness, some excitement, and of course some pride.

Finally, it will be time to take all that you have learned about yourself, relationships, and the world, and move on.

23

Preparing for crises

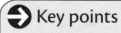
Role of crises in your recovery

Eight of the nine DSM-IV criteria for BPD imply some degree of crisis so there is no need to feel a failure when they occur. Recurrent crises are an inevitable part of the condition for most people with BPD in the earlier stages before recovery. Preparing for crises can assist in dealing with crises in a manner that restricts negative and promotes positive and productive outcomes.

Crises happen to everybody, and you are probably wondering how a crisis with all its distress can be helpful and productive. For most people with BPD, crises are an unfortunate and yet necessary part of recovery and healing. Crises are essential opportunities for learning and practising new skills, especially the skills of keeping yourself safe. In no way do we suggest that you deliberately create a crisis, in fact quite the opposite. The goal, wherever possible, is to prevent or minimize crises occurring by a growing self-awareness of the cues/triggers and chain of events (thoughts, emotions, behaviours) that lead to crisis. This self-awareness can then result in solutions that prevent or de-escalate the crisis, minimizing the negative impact of the crisis.

If crises are an inevitable part of the condition, it makes sense to plan ahead as much as possible to decrease the likelihood of negative consequences and to increase the likelihood of effective outcomes.

Accept

The first part of preparing for crises is to accept that crises will occur at least in the earlier stages of recovery. We need to move beyond our entirely understandable wishes that crises will not occur. As people-in-recovery and clinicians we all too frequently bury our heads in the sand hoping that crises will not occur, leaving us poorly prepared and less skilled when the inevitable crisis occurs.

Commitment

Having accepted that crises will inevitably occur, the next step is to commit to working on future crises. Are you able to commit, at least a little, to putting in, at least, the smallest amount of energy in preparing for future crises? We have discussed building and strengthening motivation and commitment as important ingredients of psychological change in Chapter 10.

As you no doubt well know, life for people with BPD is difficult enough in the periods between crises. In these periods, you may feel like you are just surviving, hanging in by your fingertips, and that you have absolutely nothing in the way of spare energy or surplus skills to deal with any future crisis. Unfortunately what can frequently then happen is that behaviour in the crisis makes things worse not better.

What we are going to say next is easy to say but we know through personal experience will be extremely challenging. We are suggesting that at times of crisis you will need to dig deep into yourself looking for resources that until then you may not have believed were there. People with 'nerves of steel' who do difficult anxiety-provoking things are courageous. How much more courageous then is the person with BPD whose nerves are often jangled and raw who commits to working on their crises?

Reasons for preparing for crises

To assist with your assessment as to whether it is worth committing to working on future crises, we have listed below reasons for preparing for crises:

- ◆ Increase likelihood of healthy solutions.
- ◆ Decrease likelihood of making things worse—unhealthy responses.

- ◆ Decrease likelihood of doing things impulsively that you will later regret.

- ◆ Increase self-awareness that will result in increased sense of self-effectiveness.

- ◆ To assist others' preparation for healthy supporting and helping.

- ◆ Means you are actively involved in your recovery.

- ◆ To inspire a sense of hopefulness.

As you know, when in crisis, our thinking can be muddled and we may act unwisely. If we have brainstormed possible solutions beforehand, we will be better placed to think clearly about solutions and to act wisely. As discussed in earlier chapters (Chapters 3 and 4) on diagnosis and conceptualization, impulsivity is a common feature of people with BPD. Preparing for crises tends to this problem area. You are aiming to respond to crises not like a Ferrari but like a family sedan (phrase used with permission of Jane Barrington). Increased awareness of cues/triggers, early warning signs, and the chain of events (thoughts, emotions, behaviours) leading into crisis will provide you with invaluable information to assist you in each crisis and in future crises (see Chapter 26).

Involvement of others

Family/friends and professionals will be much better positioned to support and assist you if you have previously discussed with them what you would like from them and what has worked and what has not worked for you in the past. If you are able to help them in their task of helping you, the chances are that they will feel better about helping you and better about you. It will be helpful to others to know, for example, if you have experienced advice to 'take a walk' or 'have a hot bath' as glib and minimizing of your distress. There are only so many hot baths one can take even when advice to 'have a hot bath' is supportive and helpful!

Hopefully professionals and family/friends will have communicated to you that you don't have to be suicidal in order to have contact with them. We have discussed the importance of establishing and maintaining your supportive professional and non-professional relationships in an earlier chapter (Chapter 16).

Taking charge

Being actively involved in preparing for crises will increase the likelihood of your recovery and the speed of your recovery. It is also a position of hopefulness, a topic of considerable importance discussed in greater detail earlier.

Preparing for action

Having accepted crises will happen and having made a commitment to working on future crises, you will need to take action. Any action you take is a significant step in the right direction and one that we genuinely applaud. The next step is to determine what action you might take to prepare for crises.

Later in the book, we will provide details specifically on improving distressing feelings. For the moment, however, we will focus on the preparation for crises.

Action

Written plan

Many people with BPD have commented on the value of having a crisis plan that is written down and conveniently available in places such as a wallet, purse, or by the phone. The written plan can focus attention and remind you of your wisdom. If you find you can achieve the desired results without a written plan or can do it better without a written plan—go for it—do what works best for you.

List of crisis strategies

Many people with BPD have found it helpful to list their crisis strategies, starting with the most healthy and least disruptive. The strategies you list will develop out of your growing self-awareness, especially regarding what works and what doesn't work for you. This is likely to change over time as you learn new skills and strategies.

People with BPD report how crisis planning focuses their attention on learning skills at keeping themselves safe. Crisis strategies for safety include safe people to see or telephone, safe and soothing places physically to go to, safe activities, and safe thinking.

A list of crisis strategies might also include individualized self-soothing strategies, ways of decreasing or tolerating distress, and alternatives to self-harm. The place of professional services, if relevant, will be named. To give you a tangible idea of what we have in mind we have provided below a fictitious (made up) crisis plan.

My crisis plan

This plan has been written by myself for my own use and will also be available to family/friends and clinicians to advise them how to best assist me when I am in crisis.

Advice to myself

◆ People who stay alive generally do well and get to have a satisfying life.

◆ Dealing with crises is part of my recovery.

◆ Crises are times for me to practise existing and new skills.

◆ Try my crisis strategies one at a time.

Crisis strategies

◆ Identify my emotion/s.

◆ Identify cues/triggers and early warning signs.

◆ Identify the problem—if possible solve the problem (Linehan, 2003, AA serenity prayer).

◆ If anxious and can't solve the problem try to feel better (Linehan 2003):

    ◆ use relaxation skills;

    ◆ use breathing technique if over-breathing;

    ◆ exercise;

    ◆ distract.

◆ If anxious and can't solve the problem or feel better:

    ◆ accept the anxiety—(Linehan, 2003, AA serenity prayer);

    ◆ remind myself the anxiety will lessen with time.

- If angry and can't solve the situation leading to anger:
  - walk away;
  - distract—vigorous exercise, gardening.
- If angry and can't solve the problem or feel better:
  - accept the anger—(Linehan, 2003; AA serenity prayer);
  - remind myself the anger will lessen with time;
  - angry feelings are OK (depends what I do with the feelings).
- Put on my favourite music.
- Watch a pre-recorded quality video or DVD.
- Do my self-imagery of safety.
- Telephone Jill, a safe supportive person (she will have my 'list of guidelines for others' support').
- If Jill not in—telephone Jane, another safe supportive person.
- Go to the 'safe place' in my house I have created.
- Go for a walk at the safe place for walking that I like—if daytime.
- Take quetiapine—as discussed with Dr. …—not too late to break the crisis spiral, but not too early to prevent me from practising new skills.
- Alternative to self-harm—Put hand safely in bowl of ice and reward myself afterwards if effective with visit to café.
- If none of this works—Just accept things as they are for now.
- Tel. . . . (therapist, service co-ordinator) or crisis team (out of hours).
- Respite accommodation—arrange via service/recovery co-ordinator.
- Hospital—arrange via service/recovery co-ordinator.

The statement that 'people who stay alive generally do well!' is a reminder that research and clinical experience show that generally people with BPD do get better and have satisfying lives.

The statement that crises are part of recovery is a reminder that distressing events are part of life and a reminder for you to act as much as possible in a manner that will promote your healing and recovery.

The comment to try one strategy at a time is based on feedback from people with BPD who describe being so unsettled at times of crisis that they dart from one thing to another not settling on one strategy long enough for it to work.

Individualized and evolving

An effective crisis plan will not be a meaningless glib list of theoretical possibilities but an individualized evolving plan that grows out of your unique experiences.

 Comment from Wendy

It may be hard to come to a place of being ready to develop a personal crisis plan.

Developing a crisis plan for myself in collaboration with those treating me was a lengthy process. It took me many months, if not years, to get my head around the fact that it would be useful. I had my head in the sand, always hoping that every crisis would be the last, so a crisis plan was therefore unnecessary.

Finally, having been told once too often to have a hot bath (I didn't even own a bath), I decided to give a crisis plan a go.

I used a template similar to the one above, and after lots of practice found I was more 'in control' during a crisis. People were responding more helpfully, because they had a copy of my plan, and more and more often my therapist was not involved, as the crisis resolved by my using earlier steps in the plan.

Ironically when I finally developed a crisis plan it was one of the things that helped diminish the number of crises.

24

Medication

Medications are currently almost always prescribed by a doctor (family doctor, psychiatrist, physician). However, some jurisdictions are beginning to credential prescribing, on an individual basis, to other health professionals such as psychologists and nurses.

Medication is a complex and difficult area, both for the person with BPD and for the prescribing clinician.

 Comment from Wendy

There was the temptation to blot out all feelings—meaning that I was in a Chlorpromazine 'haze'. I didn't mind this so much at first—as my bed was a very safe place—but it prevented me from learning new skills and changing.

> I will never thank enough the courageous psychiatrist who took me off what for me were overly sedating medications and dealt with the subsequent fall-out.
>
> After that I gave any medication a trial period to see if it was useful and if any intolerable side-effects diminished with time. If it met my criteria I carried on with it, if not I stopped it, in collaboration with my psychiatrist.

Why medication decisions are complex

◆ Medication might help a lot, a little, or not at all if you are depressed.

◆ Medication might help with depression but not with other BPD symptoms.

◆ There is no pill that is a sure total 'cure' for BPD.

◆ There is no medication that will help all people with BPD.

◆ Medication can reduce some symptoms for some people.

◆ Medication can make some symptoms easier to manage for some people.

◆ Some people do not benefit from medication.

◆ All medications have potential side-effects.

◆ Sometimes benefits outweigh side-effects.

◆ Sometimes side-effects outweigh benefits.

◆ Medications are unsafe when not taken as prescribed.

◆ A danger exists if being prescribed medication encourages seeing yourself as 'sick', resulting in you not taking charge of your recovery.

◆ A danger exists if medication becomes the dominant or exclusive focus of treatment rather than an adjunct to therapy, distracting you and your clinicians from the crucial skills you need to learn to have a satisfying life.

Possible effects

A brief overview of scientific research of medication treatment for BPD is covered in Chapter 9. You may want briefly to re-read this overview.

Several medications have been shown to have some effect for some people. On the other hand, there has been no trial demonstrating that any one medication is sure totally to fix or totally to cure BPD, and no medication that is a one-size-fits-all. If such a pill existed, hundreds of thousands of people with BPD around the globe would take this treatment pathway and live happy lives.

Medication often helps quite a lot if people are significantly depressed or wary of others to the extent of becoming paranoid from time to time.

Clinical experience suggests also that for some people medication reduces symptoms to a level that makes therapy more accessible, sustainable, and effective.

Sometimes peoples' impulsivity, anger, mood, and emotional stability improve on medication.

The individual benefit from any medication ranges from no benefit through moderate benefit to marked benefit.

The individual side-effects range from no side-effects through moderate side-effects to marked side-effects.

> **You and your clinicians need to weigh up possible benefits against possible side-effects of medication in deciding what medication treatment may benefit you.**

Taken together, this information suggests that a sensible pathway forward is to view taking a new medication as a trial—take it and monitor whether it helps or hinders.

Collaborate (working together towards agreed goals)

Discuss medication options in detail with your prescribing clinician, especially possible benefits and possible side-effects. Take charge of this part of your treatment as much as any other part. We encourage you to share decision-making with your prescribing clinician in a deeply collaborative manner wherever possible. This way you will be taking charge of your recovery while enabling you to benefit from expert advice from your prescribing clinician.

This pathway makes use of both you and the prescribing clinician as experts. The prescribing clinician is expert about medications including the range of possible and probable medication responses made up of benefits and side-effects and the average response that people taking the medication have had. You are expert about yourself and will be the only person with the subjective (personal) knowledge of past medication responses. You will invite the clinician to discuss your past medication effects if these are temporarily lost to your memory. For example, deterioration on stopping medication or side-effects on taking a particular medication.

You and your prescribing clinician will have to work at your respective roles. Your clinician will need to share their scientific knowledge skilfully in a way that communicates effectively to you. You will need to share your personal subjective knowledge of yourself in a manner that communicates effectively to your clinician. This is a challenging task, requiring both your and your clinician's commitment.

Trust

Effective use of medication relies on a trusting relationship between you and your prescribing clinician. Your clinician needs to trust that you will take the medication as prescribed and you need to trust that they will prescribe competently and with your best interests at heart. This does not mean that you will never have side-effects but that advantages and disadvantages of medication decision-making will have been carefully considered and discussed with you.

If you and your clinician do not see eye to eye on some matters it is your job (and theirs) to address this. It is in your interests to have the best possible relationship you can with your clinician and you need to do whatever you can to make this relationship work.

Taking medication as prescribed

Once you and your clinician have chosen a medication and decided on the dose, then it is over to you to take it as prescribed. Medication is unlikely to work if you do not take it as prescribed, and definitely will not work if you do not take it at all or overdose on it! Some clinicians will not prescribe medication for you that you have overdosed on. Others may only prescribe on a strict regimen of limited dispensing that can be a hassle for you. If you want to avoid these possibilities, take your medication as prescribed and definitely do not overdose on the medications. Overdosing on medications or stockpiling medications may undermine your relationship with your clinician as clinicians understandably do not like their prescribed medication being used intentionally harmfully or being stockpiled for possible future intentionally harmful use.

If you struggle to remember taking medication, develop your own personal reminder strategies—note on fridge, medication by toothbrush, alarm clock, watch alarm—whatever works for you.

Stopping medication

If you are having side-effects or not finding the medication that you are taking useful, contact your clinician to discuss the issue. We recommend that you do not make any unilateral decisions about stopping medication without discussing this first with your clinician. This enables you to use your clinician's expertise and also respectfully and courteously to support your clinician to support you. If you and your clinician decide to stop a medication, return the unused medication. This will cultivate trust. If the situation is urgent and your prescribing clinician is not available, contact your GP, hospital, or emergency service. These people are trained to be of assistance.

It is likely that your clinician will recommend taking any newly prescribed medication for at least a month or more (except crisis–only medications), unless side-effects are too great, before deciding on the value of the medication. Many side-effects wear off after a couple of weeks as your body adjusts to the medication and many medications rely on a satisfactory level building up in the body over a few weeks before they are fully effective.

Medication helps immediately but then stops helping

This could be a pharmacological effect but also could be a psychological effect. In being prescribed a new medication you might feel heard, understood, and supported, and be hopeful of a good medication response. This renewed sense of hope might buoy you up for a period of time.

Comment from Wendy

The excessive focus on medication and the attempts on my and my clinicians' parts to find a pharmacological 'cure' encouraged me to view myself as 'sick'—taking on the passive patient role—waiting for doctors to 'cure' me—with medication. My, and my clinicians' excessive focus on medication, biased my attention away from the more important psychological issues I critically needed to address.

My advice to you is to remember that you are the most knowledgeable person about yourself. Seek out advice about medication—and weigh up whether the benefits of the medication outweigh the side-effects—or vice versa. Work hard at establishing and maintaining a collaborative relationship with your prescribing clinician—where you can *together* explore the role of medication in complementing your other treatment

25

Hospitalization

Key points

- In this chapter we are not referring to residential *therapy*.

- Hospital can be an appropriate place of refuge, safety, and occasionally treatment, *provided it is used in the right way and at appropriate times*.

- You may or may not have had a choice over coming to hospital, but you do have choices over your behaviours and how you interact with the staff, and what the plan is from here.

- Work with staff to develop a plan.

- It is common for people to feel anxious or nervous about leaving the hospital environment.

- Survival may happen in hospital but recovery happens in the community.

Is hospital the place to be?

Acute hospital

In this chapter we are not referring to the few specialist residential therapy facilities that exist where the person with BPD lives with others with similar difficulties for several weeks or months with the express purpose of engaging in ongoing intensive therapy. Rather, we are referring in this chapter, to a stay on a psychiatric ward, usually of a hospital (acute hospital stay) where people with a wide range of different problems are treated during a short period of severe deterioration (acute deterioration).

Is hospital useful?

Yes, absolutely—hospital can be an appropriate place of refuge, safety, and occasionally treatment, *provided it is used in the right way and at appropriate times*. If you are being treated for another condition, such as severe depression or bipolar disorder, and you need to be in hospital for the best treatment, then obviously that is where you need to be. If you are at imminent risk of ending your life, then hospital can be a place where you might be better able to keep yourself safe, while you work at taking some control back and regaining your inner strength to carry on.

Difficult place to take charge of your recovery

There may be many times during the course of your recovery when you feel that you absolutely cannot cope, and want someone else to be responsible for you—hospital can seem like a golden solution to you. Unfortunately the reality is not like that. As we discussed earlier, one of the keys to healing is taking charge of your recovery, and one of the hardest places in the world to do that is in hospital.

Hospital can become a place where you feel safe not to have to face the realities of life outside. It is easy in the hospital environment to stop taking charge, letting others take charge, which feeds those beliefs that you are inadequate and unable to cope with life.

In hospital it can often appear that there is no need to maintain even a thin veneer of coping, and suddenly the things you were managing in your life, even if it was only the basics like getting out of bed each day, and cooking for yourself, can quickly fall away, making you feel worse, 'sicker', 'proving' to you that you really cannot manage your life.

Frequent hospital admissions can lead to a downward spiral of hopelessness, only serving to prove to you that you are getting 'sicker' and 'sicker'.

Different staff

The hospital professionals will probably be part of a large team of nurses and doctors and possibly psychologists, social workers, and occupational therapists, and hospital professionals are often different from those treating you in the community. External consistency and continuity, which you so badly need to balance your internal turmoil, can be sadly lacking, making your internal world even more chaotic. When you are at your most vulnerable, being in hospital may mean getting differing opinions and ideas on what you 'should' be doing. You may get different responses and attitudes from different staff about yourself, whether you should be in hospital or not, what you should be doing for yourself, and how much staff time you should have.

Recovery happens in the community

For recovery to happen in the community and for you to stay out of hospital, you will require effective treatment being available to you in the community. If this treatment is not available, it might mean that you are in hospital more often.

It has been our universal experience that while being in hospital might help people survive in the short term, recovery happens in the community. This makes perfect sense if you think about it. To recover, you need to learn, practise, and become effective at using skills in the world that you want to live in. Generally, hospitals, for the reasons described previously, are often counterproductive in assisting you to learn the long-term skills required for success in your world. Survival may happen in the hospital, but recovery happens in the community.

Client-controlled hospitalization

Some services offer short, planned 'client-controlled' admissions. A client-controlled admission can occur when you and your treating clinicians have proactively negotiated an agreement that a brief stay in hospital (say 48–96 hours) for respite or time out might be helpful. This will be part of your treatment plan and, because the plan involves so many people, will best be documented. You and others engaged in the plan relate to you as a responsible intelligent person who will use the plan wisely. You do not have to be in 'crisis' or at imminent risk to use a client-controlled admission—in fact, a sense that things are deteriorating and a wish to prevent a crisis can be a really appropriate way to use a client-controlled admission. It allows you to gain the support you require, without any need for things to escalate, power struggles, or a requirement to 'prove' how much you need to be in hospital.

Your proactively negotiated client-controlled agreement is likely to include how long your stay will be, what the likely goals are for the time in hospital, who will provide transport to and from hospital, what the roles of hospital staff are, and, if relevant what the contingencies (what will happen next) will be of self-harm in hospital.

Some clinicians and hospitals are of the opinion that self-harming during a client-controlled admission shows that the admission is not being useful, and is a criterion for discharge. Others state that so long as self-harm is private, cleaned up by the person-in-recovery, and not requiring medical attention, it should be viewed neutrally by staff. Self-harm *per se* is not usually seen as a reason to lengthen the duration of a client-controlled admission.

If you are too much at risk to leave hospital in the designated time it might be that a client-controlled admission is not for you and you will need to return to a traditional clinician-controlled admission procedure.

I am in hospital—now what?

You may end up in hospital in a proactively planned way (client-controlled admission) or you might end up in hospital in an unplanned way due to imminent concerns you have or others have for your safety (acute admission).

Acute admission

An acute admission refers to an admission that was not planned ahead of time but happens because of imminent concerns about your safety or occasionally the safety of others.

Stop and take a deep breath

Hospital might or might not be where you want to be, but you are here now and you have support to keep yourself safe.

Take back some control

You may or may not have had a choice over coming to hospital, but you do have choices over your behaviours and how you interact with the staff, and what the plan is from here.

Plan

Work with the staff to develop a plan (may be called a hospital or care plan). It will be similar to your community plan, but covering the specific time you are in hospital and may include:

◆ Brief history (1–2 paragraphs) to save you from needing to tell your story repeatedly.

◆ Your goals while in hospital (hopefully these will be the same as the staff's goals, but, if not, a statement of their goals too).

◆ List of what you believe you will find helpful from staff.

- List of what you believe you will find unhelpful from staff.

- Expectations that you have of staff.

- Expectations staff have of you.

- Support to help you meet staff expectations.

- Consequences if you do not meet these expectations.

- When discharge will occur, if this is pre-determined.

- What if anything that needs to happen for discharge to occur.

Work on your goals (with staff if applicable)

Remember that taking charge will be a key to recovery, so the sooner you can do things for yourself, the better.

Examine what led you to be in hospital

Examine step by step what led you to be in hospital with a view to solutions to the problem, if possible. If you are feeling reasonably OK, work with the staff to see if there were any points at which the chain of events could have been interrupted or changed and how this crisis could be stopped from happening another time.

Distress tolerance skills

Where you can't solve the problem, you will need to work on how you can feel better even though the problem still exists. Staff can help you here, and both you and they might draw from DBT's distress tolerance skills. If you are familiar with DBT, use all of the DBT skills that you know about that have been useful for you.

Leaving hospital

You may be tempted to do things and behave in ways that serve to encourage staff to delay your discharge. Ask yourself what will be the wisest ways for you to proceed and use all the effective skills you have to advance your recovery. It is common for people to feel anxious or nervous about leaving the hospital environment.

> **Survival may happen in hospital, but recovery happens in the community**

Client-controlled admission

Congratulate yourself

◆ You have stated what you needed in a healthy assertive way.

◆ You are caring for yourself by taking a few days time-out.

Plan

◆ If you do not already have one, work with the staff to develop a hospital plan (see above, and template below).

◆ Structure your time (e.g. rest, working on goals, eating, support).

◆ Work on your goals, examine what led you to be in hospital, use distress tolerance skills and plan for leaving hospital (as above in acute admission).

The following template serves as a catalyst (method) for you to include and remove whatever will work best for you in your unique situation.

Template for hospital plan

Brief description of myself (include strengths)

Recent events (cues/triggers, chain of events)

My goals while in hospital

I find the following helpful: e.g. having someone to talk to, journal writing, walking, distress tolerance exercises

I find the following unhelpful: e.g. noise, being told what to do, agreements not kept

If I self-harm (insert actions that will occur)

I will be discharged on (insert date)

Signed:

_____   _____   _____
Person-in-recovery   Community key worker   Hospital key worker

---

Comment from Wendy

In the 10 years prior to my recovery I had in excess of 50 admissions to various psychiatric units, some brief, but the majority lasting weeks to several months. I can now see that this was a destructive path, only serving to 'prove' to me that I really was helpless and hopeless. It was necessary, but not easy for me, to detach from my destructive 'love affair' with being in hospital to learn how to stop 'limping', start walking, and take charge of my life again.

Section 3

Recovery specifics

In Section 3, we outline some specific strategies that you might find helpful. A comprehensive discussion of all possible skills is beyond the scope of this book. Instead, we have selected skills that are practical and of recognized value in everyday life and have been helpful to Wendy and/or others in tending to distress, dealing with emotions, having relationships with self and others, and taking action with skilful behaviours that have improved quality of life. Some of the specific strategies will be sufficient as written in this book while others serve just to highlight areas for discussion and exploration with your therapist. Many or most of the skills can be useful for all of us whether we have BPD or not, as they are skills for living. Other skills are more specifically targeted for people with BPD. You may consider this section like a toolbox that can be revisited many times.

26

Is it our awareness that makes a difference? (Self-reflection, chain analysis, and mindfulness)

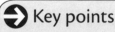 Key points

- Self-reflection of current experience requires us rapidly to shift our focus from full immersion in the experience to a position of stepping back just enough to allow for some degree of watching ourselves and self-reflection, and then to throw ourselves back into the experience, and so forth.

- Self-reflection enables us to take ownership of our experiences.

- Self-reflection is a psychological skill that requires practice.

- The aim of the chain analysis is to identify problems in the chain of events that occurred and then to explore solutions that will better prepare us the next time we are in a similar position.

- Solution planning is the development of a 'toolbox' of skills to allow us to embrace alternative healthier actions.

> ◆ Doing chain analyses of successful skilful behaviours can provide a balance if the going gets too tough just doing chain analyses of problem behaviours.
>
> ◆ Chain analyses can be a very effective recovery tool for the rest of our lives.
>
> ◆ Mindfulness is a practice of paying attention leading to awareness.

Self-reflection

Self-reflection is a term used to describe the capacity to monitor our own thoughts, emotions, and behaviours directly. This 'psychological mindedness' involves being able to think about thinking, think about feeling, and think about behaviour. It also involves feeling about thinking, feeling about emotions, and feeling about behaviour. This enables us to have a sense of ownership of our own thoughts, emotions, and behaviours.

Self-reflection is a focus of attention for all psychological therapies, to the best of our knowledge. Self-reflection may be a primary and dominant goal of some therapies. Other therapies will utilize self-reflection as a means of achieving goals such as behaviour change. Whatever therapy you are in, it is well recognized that the capacity to step back and reflect upon our internal world and the world external to us is an important and valuable psychological skill. Psychodynamic* and mentalization*-based therapies will encourage your alertness to your inner world including how this manifests in the relationship with your therapist. In psychodynamic* therapies, the therapy relationship is used as a vehicle for learning self-awareness, which in turn provides us with the skills to deal with our lives more effectively.

In the course of life, you will have many experiences. Therapy will encourage your reflection upon these experiences especially the more intense experiences. If the experience takes place during the therapy session and/or is about the therapy relationship, you will be encouraged to enter into the experience fully and wholeheartedly, subject to this being productive.

You will be encouraged to reflect upon all experiences both during and after the experience. Reflecting upon a recent past experience is different from reflecting upon the experience while it is happening. Reflecting upon experience after the experience has the advantage of being a slower process as the emotional intensity will have usually waned.

On the other hand, reflecting upon current experience has the advantage of the experience and details of the experience being immediately available to reflection. Being able to reflect upon current experience is a challenging task but one that has the potential to change and revolutionize our lives. If we are able both to experience fully and to reflect upon the experience as it is happening, we will have a vast amount of information available to us to assist our effective decision-making in the moment. When we are able to string together a series of effective decisions we will be able to influence the course of our lives positively.

Self-reflection of current experience requires us rapidly to shift our focus from full immersion in the experience to a position of stepping back just enough to allow for some degree of watching ourselves and self-reflection, and then to throw ourselves back into the experience, and so forth. This gives us a self-reflection loop inside the experience enabling us to affect the outcome of the situation (Fig. 26.1).

We need to be able to identify the need for stepping back, take charge, step back, and be sure to not step back too far. If we step back too far we lose connection with the experience, resulting in an overly intellectual and unemotive position or even emotional numbness.

You (and your therapist) will be repeatedly encouraging self-reflection by asking questions such as, 'What am I thinking? What am I feeling?' You will be repeatedly standing back to ask yourself, 'What do I make of this experience?' You will become expert at unravelling your experience, opening the experience up for analysis.

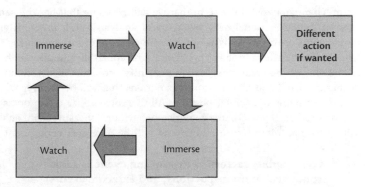

Fig 26.1 Self-reflective loop inside the experience enabling us to influence the outcome. We wish to acknowledge the ideas from DBT (Linehan), mentalization (Bateman, Fonagy, Holmes), and transtheoretical approach (Prochaska, Norcross and DiClimente) in our development of this figure'.

Self-reflection enables us to take ownership of our experiences. This ownership enables us to influence our experience including regulating our behaviour and emotions. Sometimes professionals use the term 'mentalizing*' to describe self-reflection processes that also include our reflection on the world of other people. Reflection on the world of others enables us to know their world better, resulting in increased capacity for empathy. This will improve our capacity for social reciprocity, leading to improved relationships.

Self-reflection is a psychological skill that requires practice. Just like physical training gets our muscles fit and able to carry out tasks we could not previously do, so it is with self-reflection. We need to practise and train our minds to become fit and skilled at self-reflection. Self-reflection is particularly relevant for people who tend, for better or worse, to be emotionally intense and inclined to act too rapidly or impulsively.

Chain analysis

From the range of CBT language, we have chosen to use DBT language, as this will be familiar to readers in DBT treatment. We wish to acknowledge Linehan and Behavioural Tech for the terms 'chain analysis, problem analysis, solution analysis, vulnerability factors, prompting event, links, problem behaviour, consequences and repair', and for the ideas (along with other CBT clinicians) on which this section on chain analysis is based.

Another way of monitoring ourselves and the world around us is via chain analysis (Fig. 26.2).

The term 'chain analysis' is the term that we will be using that has the same meaning as 'functional analysis', 'behavioural analysis', and 'problem and solution analysis'. A chain analysis outlines the chain of events and links that led up to and came after a problem behaviour (and sometimes solution behaviour). The aim of the chain analysis is to identify problems in the chain of events that occurred and then to explore solutions that will better prepare us the next time we are in a similar position. All therapies utilize this process in one way or another. If you are in a cognitive-behavioural therapy, chain analyses will be formal, often written down and will be a central component of

> **Vulnerability factors ⇒ Prompting event ⇒ Links**
> **(thoughts, emotions, actions, and external events)**
> **⇒ Problem behaviour ⇒ Consequneces ⇒ Repair**

Figure 26.2 Chain analysis.

treatment. Other therapies will also be interested in the sequence of internal and external events that led to problems or successful solutions.

Problem behaviour

The problem behaviour is anything you (and your therapist) define as a problem—it may be self-harm, using substances, yelling at children, assault, gambling, unsafe sex, numbing out, dissociating, binge eating, or deliberate vomiting. Urges to problematic behaviours can also be the subject of chain analysis, e.g. urges to suicide, self-harm, use substances, gamble, leave therapy, etc. Be very specific about exactly what the problem behaviour was and when it happened. Starting a formal chain analysis with the problem behaviour keeps us focused on the purpose of the chain analysis, which is to identify problems and solutions.

Defining urges as targets of intervention can be really valuable as it encourages awareness of links in the chain of events when it is still possible to reflect and do something differently. For example, early warning signs of numbing out can result in us preventing dissociation. Early warning signs of leaving therapy can prevent the impulsive leaving of therapy.

Vulnerability factors

Explore the events that made you vulnerable or predisposed you to problem behaviours. Vulnerability factors are ones that leave us susceptible to problem behaviour. Were you tired, sleep deprived, physically unwell, having money worries or premenstrual symptoms? The possibilities are endless. As you do more and more chain analyses you will begin to see patterns, and can then look at trying to reduce vulnerability factors where this is possible. For example, tending to painful medical and dental conditions will maximize health and decrease pain, leaving us more resilient (hardy) to face the challenges that life throws at us and more resilient in the face of prompting events. In the same way improving our sleep will leave us more refreshed and resilient to face the challenges and to enjoy the pleasures of the day.

Prompting event

Look hard for what pushed your buttons enough to start the process of thoughts, emotions, and actions that led to the problem behaviour. Once we can identify a pattern of prompting events, we can then decide whether it will be wise or unwise to try to avoid this particular prompting event in the future.

Sometimes it will be wise to avoid the prompting event. Avoiding being near alcohol wherever possible is wise for almost all people who are early in their recovery from alcohol problems. On other occasions it will be impossible to avoid the prompting event. Such an example might be when night-time is a prompting event.

For other events, we will wisely and deliberately choose to not avoid the prompting event, so that we can practise and get better skilled in the face of the prompting event. This will leave us more resilient as life is full of potential prompting events. An example might be being cued/triggered by interaction with men. Often we cannot control prompting events but we can learn to plan solutions for when the prompting event occurs. Of course, once we get skilled at dealing with previously triggering events the events will cease triggering us.

Links (thoughts, emotions, actions, and external events)

Thoughts, emotions, and actions interact with one another, which can lead to more thoughts, emotions, and actions, accentuating the distress leading to the problem behaviour. Solutions may include putting in place more effective ways of thinking and acting that will lead to skilful actions in future to break the chain. Solution planning is the development of a 'toolbox' of skills to allow us to embrace alternative healthier actions.

Consequences

Often the consequences of problem behaviour can become a new prompting event, creating a never ending downward spiral. Recognizing and naming the consequences can be a good start to breaking this cycle.

Repair

Our problem behaviours may have a negative impact not only upon ourselves but also on others. If this is the case, see whether you can make some repair or some way to make amends.

Vulnerability factors	Problem analysis	Solution analysis
Prompting event		
Links (thoughts, emotions, actions, and external events)		
Problem behaviour		
Consequences for self		
For others		
Repair		

This figure is based on ideas of Marsha M. Linehan, Behavioral Tech LLC, and Seth Axelrod.

Fig 26.3 Chain analysis

You might want to write solutions in a different colour. An alternative way of doing the chain analysis is to write the thoughts, emotions, and actions down on a piece of paper, joining them with linking arrows.

Comment from Wendy

I really disliked chain analyses when I was first introduced to them. It was not easy for me publicly to explore my problems in exquisite detail. I found chain analyses frequently unpleasant as they often led to distressing emotions. I did them reluctantly because it was expected of me, and if ever I could get out of doing one I did. However, despite my initial reluctance I did lots, and began to discover that my chain of thoughts, emotions, and behaviours often followed similar patterns with similar outcomes. I began to recognize these patterns and started identifying parts of the pattern/s earlier on in the chain when they reoccurred. In time I learned healthier solutions that I would practise so that I could put these into action when I identified going down familiar pathways.

Hurdles

If we have not done this type of thing before, it can be unfamiliar and very challenging. By their very nature, chain analyses are usually designed to high-light problems that we have. This can be very hard. None of us particularly likes our faults being scrutinized and known to others. So, be gentle and compassionate with yourself as you engage in this courageous and honest exploration. Doing chain analyses of successful skilful behaviours can provide a balance if the going gets too tough just doing chain analyses of problem behaviours.

The rewards of chain analyses may not be immediately apparent; however, the rewards of persisting can be considerable. With practice the process can become second nature and a skill we can find ourselves using naturally and informally in our everyday lives. Chain analyses can be a very effective recovery tool for the rest of our lives.

Mindfulness/attention control

Another way of improving awareness of ourselves and the world around us is mindfulness/attention control.

Have you ever found yourself saying about yourself or others, 'That was mind-less'. Being mindful or attentive is the opposite of mindless.

All therapies, to the best of our knowledge, encourage being attentive to our-selves and the world we live in, so as to become increasingly aware. Mindfulness or attention control is a pathway to awareness. This awareness provides the information to clarify our emotions, identity, goals, and values, and for formal or informal chain analyses enabling us to identify problems and guide our future healthy decision-making (solution analysis).

The term 'mindfulness' is sometimes used as a way of describing the practice of paying attention or concentration and does not require any religious or spiritual affiliations, although it can be integrated into religious or spiritual life should you want. Mindfulness can be part of everyday life or can be practised more formally via attention control, contemplation, meditation, yoga, and other classes. As with most skills, the more we practice, the better we will get.

Mindfulness has now earned its current place in mainstream Western psychological practices. DBT, which has a strong base of research evidence of effectiveness for treating people with BPD, is strongly influenced by mindfulness practice. Attention control/mindfulness has also been shown to be effective in treating people with chronic physical pain and in preventing relapse in people who are prone to repeated episodes of depression.

It is not feasible for us to be able to tell you in this book how to practise mindfulness/attention control. If you are interested in mindfulness/attention control, discuss your interest with your therapist to see whether it can or can't be integrated into your recovery by your therapist directly or via a class that may be run, for example, at a community centre.

 Comment from Wendy

I used to consider mindfulness to be an 'out there' Eastern religious practice that was for people who looked and behaved differently from me.

I thought that you had to sit silently and motionlessly for long periods of time. With this view, I could not see how it could possibly be part of my life.

I did not realize that mindfulness is just about paying attention—no more and no less, and that we all use mindfulness skills in our everyday life. For example, paying attention to listening to our friends or paying attention to a mundane activity such as washing the dishes. One of my favourites is cooking. I can be amazed at the number of textures, sights, smells, and sounds involved.

I took some mindfulness classes and, while like any other skill it required regular practice, was surprised at the simplicity.

Mindfulness can be practised anywhere, anytime, and for as long or as short as you choose, and can be an incredibly good way of settling intense emotions, or letting time pass so the emotions settle themselves.

27

Is it what we do that makes a difference?

> ## Key points

- ◆ The challenge for all of us is to behave skilfully and effectively even when we are feeling distressed.

- ◆ For many of us changing our behaviour in the short term can have the effect of improving our distress and changing our emotions for the better.

- ◆ To feel better in the long term we also need to put in place behaviours that will increase the likelihood of us achieving our long-term goals.

- ◆ What will be of relevance to one person might not be of relevance to another.

- ◆ As human beings we are motivated to fill our lives with activities that we experience as rewarding. Rewarding activities might be pleasurable, purposeful, or meaningful.

- ◆ It is important that we maintain or develop lives of relevance despite our distress as lives of relevance can build the structures that will decrease our distress long term.

Behaviour, action, doing

It is easy for us to be skilful in our behaviours when we are feeling happy and content. However, we are all more vulnerable to acting unskilfully when we are feeling distressed. This is referred to as 'mood-dependent behaviour', i.e. our behaviour depends on our mood at the time. The challenge for all of us is to behave skilfully and effectively even when we are feeling distressed.

For many of us changing our behaviour in the short term can have the effect of improving our distress and changing our emotions for the better. We need to put in place behaviours that increase the chances of this happening. This will include individualized pleasurable, purposeful, and meaningful behaviours. You will need to reflect on what works best for you. Many people with BPD have difficulty deliberately doing things for themselves that are pleasurable, feeling undeserving of such activities. If this applies to you, we encourage you to reflect upon your view considering the alternative view that having fun and looking after oneself can be healthy and have a beneficial effect on those around you also.

Short-term day-to-day purposeful activities such as washing the dishes, gardening, cooking, and cleaning achieve something and help many of us feel a little satisfied. At the end of the activity we gain the benefit of the activity, such as clean dishes, and also the satisfaction of doing something successfully, however small. On a really difficult day we can remind ourselves that we can still be successful at doing some small things.

Meaningful activity usually refers to something a little deeper than washing the dishes for example, and that tends to bring out human qualities about ourselves that we value. Activities may include doing something kind for someone, working, learning a new skill, creative activities (e.g. painting, music), or engaging in prayer or other spiritual or religious activity.

To feel better in the long term we also need to put in place behaviours that will increase the likelihood of us achieving our long-term goals. This may include building our relationships with family and friends and building our work or work-related activities. As we start achieving these types of goals we understandably will feel better about ourselves, our lives, and the world.

Life of relevance

What do we mean by the phrase 'life of relevance'? We all will have different ideas of what constitutes for ourselves a life of relevance. What will be of relevance to one person might not be of relevance to another. Also what we consider relevant might well change as we move through life.

Among numerous activities, it might be relevant for a child to play or to go to school, a young adult to explore, or study, or work, an adult to befriend, parent, or work, and an older person to retire, work, or travel. There are optimal levels of activity. Too much activity and we might feel stressed, too little and our lives may feel insufficiently full.

The type of activity will also determine the quality of our lives. As human beings we are motivated to fill our lives with activities that we experience as rewarding. Rewarding activities will be pleasurable, purposeful, or meaningful, and will be determined also by our values and identity. We have discussed these issues in other chapters on identity and values, pleasure, relationships with ourselves, others, and something larger than ourselves (the latter being the language that some people use to describe their spiritual experience).

If you are working full-time or parenting young children, your life will be busy. If not, you might engage in relevant activities that include study at educational institutions, study at local community centre courses, part-time work, voluntary work, community service, joining a club, supporting a sports team, growing a garden, developing a new skill such as cooking or computers, and other activities of relevance for you.

It is important that we maintain or develop lives of relevance despite our distress as lives of relevance can build the structures that will decrease our distress long term. We encourage you to explore how you might fill your days with relevance as part of your recovery.

Comment from Wendy

A good friend once said to me that a contented life requires enough happy moments. For some of us, sometimes, recalling past happy moments when we are distressed can be tricky. One way to remember happy moments is a 'positive book', otherwise known as a self-soothing journal or a happy book. This is your own personal journal that could be very precious to you, as it was to me. Depending on your financial situation, you could buy a large notepad or a fancy journal. You could decorate a shoe box or buy a gift box or photo box that fits your journal into it, plus glue, felt tips, stickers, and scissors.

During each day you could take a note of the small 'high' points—maybe someone commented on your tidy house, maybe you enjoyed coffee with a friend, maybe the cat cuddled up close, or maybe you were pleased with the way you handled a situation. Whatever the little positives are in each day; take time to note them down in your journal. The idea of the journal is to remind yourself of anything that lifts your mood.

Things that were helpful to me included:

- pressed leaves or flowers from a special place
- photos of people that I valued
- cards from friends with personal messages in them
- achievements I was proud of
- ticket stubs from a movie I enjoyed, or a sports match or concert I attended
- postcards of a destination I love
- quotes that inspired me
- a joke that made me laugh
- an email that was positive

Anything else that inspires you.

This book can be a reminder of small past positive aspects of your life and can encourage you to notice positive events in the present, today.

28

Is it what we think that makes a difference?

> ### ➜ Key points
>
> ◆ There is hope—we can rewrite the self-talk script.
>
> ◆ A thought is just a thought. That is, it is not necessarily a fact. It may be a fact, but it may not be a fact.
>
> ◆ Ineffective self-talk does not belong in your future—and it may well have not even been accurate in the past.
>
> **JCOB (Acronym developed by Sandy Byers Evitt and group members)**
>
> ◆ **J**umping to conclusions—this type of thought pattern occurs when we don't wait to hear a full explanation or to get enough information to make an accurate assessment of a situation. We *jump to a conclusion* without sufficient evidence.
>
> ◆ **C**atastrophizing—this occurs when we assume the worst possible outcome from a situation without giving thought or weight to other possible outcomes.
>
> ◆ **O**vergeneralizing—this occurs when we excessively generalize a response to a single negative event into other areas of our lives.
>
> ◆ **B**lack and white thinking—when we engage in *black or white thinking*, we only see two options. Often these two options are *all-good* or *all-bad* and often involve judgements about ourselves and others.

Self-talk

Self-talk is a term that is used for the things we think and say to ourselves all the time, often without even being aware of it. It is our internal dialogue. It is our running commentary of our views of ourselves, our lives, and the world, and exists in the thinking part of ourselves.

Much of our self-talk is embedded in our psyche from a very young age. People (including parents, family, friends, and teachers) and life experiences influence our beliefs and opinions about ourselves and the world. Our core ways of thinking, our core beliefs become automatic: so automatic that we do not reassess the factual validity of our thoughts and beliefs in the present. Were you ever told, 'Children should be seen and not heard?' Unless this statement was countered with positive statements and lots of opportunities to be heard and valued, you are likely to have developed an idea that your opinion was not worth anything.

In later life, this same self-talk may recur—you may have a brilliant idea at a meeting, but you will be saying to yourself, 'My ideas and opinions are worthless'. This is ineffective self-talk, and can be damaging if not challenged. Clues to ineffective self-talk may be words such as 'must' and 'should'. Watch out for messages that are critical about yourself in particular and check them for accuracy and relevance to your adult life.

> **There is hope—we can rewrite the script**

A thought is just a thought

Self-talk can be harmful and ineffective or helpful and effective. Reflect for a moment that a thought is just a thought. That is, it is not necessarily a fact. It may be a fact, but it may not be a fact. If we have a thought, 'I can't do this', it is just a thought. Whether we can do the activity or not remains unanswered and will need to be explored. Identifying a thought as just a thought allows us to reassess the factual validity of the thought. In the example used, it enables us to consider doing the activity despite having the thought, 'I can't do this'. This might result in us being able to do the activity, thereby changing our perception of ourselves and our future. Our thinking might become, 'Maybe, I can do this'. We will have changed a hopeless ineffective way of thinking into a hopeful effective way of thinking.

Effective self-talk

Self-talk can become so automatic that we often have little or no conscious awareness of what we are saying to ourselves. Try spending some time thinking about the messages you give to yourself—think about where they came from and whether they are still useful or appropriate now. Try thinking of some effective self-talk you can replace the ineffective self-talk with. An hour of not yelling at the children could lead to a change of self-talk from, 'I am always yelling at my children' to 'I often but not always yell at my children' and if applicable to, 'I sometimes yell at my children'. A small success in any area of your life could lead you to say to yourself, 'I can be successful'.

Changing your self-talk is not necessarily an easy process and needs to be given your attention. Start out by simply noticing what you say to yourself, and then one at a time, look for evidence to see whether that statement is still valid, and, if not, replace it. Also take notice when things go well and give yourself credit. Each time you find you are saying the same ineffective things to yourself, challenge them gently, and your self-talk can transform to a helpful and positive tool.

Ineffective self-talk does not belong in your future—and it may well have not even been accurate in the past

Ineffective thinking

We all have some ineffectiveness in our thinking, where our thoughts, although seemingly rational and logical, are actually based on incorrect assumptions. Ineffective thoughts are often so habitual that they slip by unnoticed. Recognizing our thoughts as thoughts not facts is very hopeful as we can change our thoughts.

JCOB

So, how do we recognize ineffective thinking? JCOB is an acronym for some common examples of ineffective thinking that might help us learn to recognize our ineffective thinking.

◆ **J**umping to conclusions

◆ **C**atastrophizing

◆ **O**vergeneralizing

◆ **B**lack and white thinking.

Jumping to conclusions

This type of thought pattern occurs when we don't wait to hear a full explanation or to get enough information to make an accurate assessment of a situation. We *jump to a conclusion* without sufficient evidence.

We can challenge this by stopping and taking a breath before we panic or overreact and think to ourselves, 'Do I have all the information I need?' 'What other information do I need before I can make a wise evaluation of the meaning?'

'Mind reading' is a form of *jumping to conclusions*. Have you ever been asked to attend a meeting and immediately thought, 'What have I done wrong'? This is an example of *jumping to a conclusion* without the information we need to develop an informed opinion. The person inviting us may be wishing to congratulate us, seek out our valuable opinion, or discuss a pay rise with us, and our angst will have been fruitless.

When somebody yawns, we might *jump to a conclusion* that they find us boring, when in fact they may be sleep deprived, may have had a long hard day, or they may be someone that yawns a lot whoever they are with.

We (Roy and Wendy) do a lot of teaching and we are alert to people yawning as a possible sign that the teaching is not stimulating enough. If one person only out of 30 yawns, then we assume the evidence for the teaching being very boring is low. If 10 out of 30 people are yawning, the evidence is now large that something is amiss. We now need to explore whether the room is too hot, it is too long since the last tea break, too long since a food break, too late in the day, or whether it is our teaching that is the problem. We have to remind ourselves not to *jump to conclusions* and seek out further information (evidence) for any one assumption.

Catastrophizing

This occurs when we assume the worst possible outcome from a situation without giving thought or weight to other possible outcomes.

This is the opposite of hopefulness, where we look 'for a favourable outcome within the realm of possibilities' (Clarke, 2003). Decreasing *catastrophic thinking* and increasing hopefulness is important because we are more likely to feel better while being realistically hopeful. Being hopeful has been shown to improve our energy to take action that then results in greater likelihood of achieving our goals.

If we are *catastrophizing*, we will also have a belief that what has happened or will happen will be unbearable and that, 'I will not be able to stand it'.

We can challenge *catastrophic thinking* and invite realistic hopefulness by asking ourselves, 'Am I thinking the worst?', 'What is the likelihood or probability of this occurring?', 'Could I survive if that outcome occurred?' or where appropriate saying to ourselves, 'If the worst happens, I will not like it, however, I will be able to stand it'.

Most of us have been in a situation where we are meeting someone and the other person is delayed. Do we immediately presume we have been stood up because they do not like us, or that they have been involved in a dreadful motor vehicle accident, or do we entertain the possibility that they may have had a flat tyre, or the babysitter was late?

Overgeneralizing

This occurs when we excessively generalize a response to a single negative event into other areas of our lives (*overgeneralize*). For example, after a setback do we say, 'See, I am useless at everything'. We may overestimate the degree to which future negative events will take place on the basis of a current negative event? There is a filtering of the event so that we focus on negatives while discounting positives.

We may excessively personalize things attributing a disproportionate amount of responsibility to ourselves. For example, 'I am useless at keeping friends, if only I had made more of a special effort, my friend would not have moved town'.

Do our language, thoughts, and self-talk frequently contain words like 'all', 'every', 'no one', 'never', 'everybody', or 'nobody'? These words often indicate that we are *overgeneralizing* as it is very uncommon for example that, 'good things *never* happen' '*all* men are …', or '*all* women are …'. Changing these words to 'frequently, sometimes, maybe, or occasionally' can assist us living in the world with greater lightness.

Black and white thinking

Alternative ways that you may have heard *black and white thinking* described are *all-or-nothing, absolutist, or dichotomous thinking*. When we engage in *black or white thinking*, we only see two options. Often these two options are *all-good or all-bad* and often involve judgements about ourselves and others.

The people we like probably have some features that we do not like that much, and people we dislike will probably have some redeeming features.

Black and white thinking often involves us being harshly critical of ourselves. This harsh self-judgement will keep our energy for change low. It is hard for anyone to get motivated when they are being told off and scolded. Try changing, for example, 'I am useless at everything' to 'I can … (e.g. cook, run a home, listen well), and 'Nobody ever does anything for me' to, 'Jill, rang me, John listened to me'.

When evaluating a situation we may only see two choices—the *absolute* right choice and the *absolute* wrong choice, when in reality most choices have advantages and disadvantages. We might believe that there is only one right way to do things. In actual fact there are hundreds of shades between black and white, and often there are many solutions or ways of looking at a situation.

How many ways do you think there are to make an omelette? We can think of about six ways, all probably likely to turn out a good tasty omelette, even if the method was not the one we previously would have seen as the right way. Also, if we cooked six omelettes in different ways and gave them to 100 readers, I am sure we would see a wide range of people's preferences—thank goodness!

We need to try avoiding the *all-or-nothing* route. If we can't clean our house from top to bottom, including the ceilings and every window, it can still be worthwhile washing the dishes or tidying up the lounge.

When you see the range of possibilities in situations, you will know that you have taken a giant step in your recovery. It takes practice to look for the range of possibilities and options. We wish you well with your practice.

29

Is it what we feel that makes a difference?

➡ Key points

- Four of the basic emotions described are fear, happiness, anger, and sadness.

- Emotions have important functions—they provide information about ourselves and our environment.

- Emotions are neither right nor wrong—they just are.

- Emotions are one part of ourselves—they are not the total of us.

- A primary emotion is an emotion that we experience in response to an internal or external event.

- A secondary emotion is an emotion we can have about the primary emotion on the basis of our self-critical beliefs about the primary emotion.

- Secondary emotions are often more problematic than are primary emotions.

- The way to deal with distressing secondary emotions is to accept our primary emotions.

Emotions

Emotions can be confusing, especially if we are not used to experiencing or recognizing them. Some people with BPD are aware of intense emotions but the range of awareness of emotions is restricted to one grouping of emotions such as angry emotions. One person with BPD described their mechanism of dealing with emotions as being like a damaged floodgate that is either completely closed or completely open, with no in-between (Bartels and Crotty, 1998). Your emotions may seem like they are either all locked in or spilling out everywhere, distressing you and perhaps those around you. It doesn't need to be like this.

We describe four of the basic emotions, with each having several variations and thousands of minuscule steps on a scale depending on their intensity. The four basic emotions described are fear, happiness, anger, and sadness.

Not uncommonly two emotions can be felt in a very short time in response to the same cue. Think of a ride on a roller-coaster. It is common for emotions in this situation to include both exhilaration (happiness) and terror (fear) shortly after one another.

Emotions have important functions

Emotions can be useful gauges and have important functions. When we are presented with a situation, our brains quickly evaluate the situation, comparing it with past experience and reacting with an emotion. Emotions provide information about ourselves and our environment, and are essential for effective decision-making.

> **Emotions provide information about ourselves and our environment**

Fear and anger can warn us of impending danger and cause us to move or avoid a situation, sadness can tell us that what we are sad about is something of value to us, and happiness encourages us to recreate the situation resulting in happiness.

If our lives have been one where almost all emotions have been distressing, it will be understandable that we might try to bury or avoid experiencing our emotions. If this is the case, discuss this with your therapist, exploring how you might find a way to begin to experience emotions early on when they are small and not overwhelming and when you can have a decent chance at using the information from your emotions to generate effective functioning and cultivating of desirable emotions.

Emotions just are

Emotions are neither right nor wrong—they just are. Whether experiencing an emotion is helpful or harmful depends on how we act in response to the emotion. For example, it will be unhelpful if our anger results in us choosing to assault a person and we end up in prison, but helpful and effective if our anger leads us to choose effectively to avoid people who are unsafe. Sexual feelings can be harmful if they lead us to unsafe sex or helpful if they lead us to pleasure. Feelings of wanting human connection can harmfully lead us to getting together with people who use us or can lead us to making satisfying relationships.

Distress happens: how we behave will be what is important

Extreme distress can result in our choosing behaviours designed to decrease the pain and distress in the short term that end up making things even worse for ourselves, i.e. mood-dependent behaviour. Emotions themselves, even distressing emotions, are not necessarily a problem. Our task is to act skilfully and effectively in accordance with our personal values despite distressing feelings or moods.

Our emotions belong to us

Nobody can know for sure what another human being is feeling. It is important for us to tell people what we are feeling if we want to be sure that they know what we are feeling.

It is equally important that we recognize that while we can make an informed guess at how somebody else is feeling by their facial and body posture, we can't be sure unless they tell us. So, if it is important that we know what someone else is feeling, it might be that we need to ask them.

If we have pleasing emotions around another person, we can choose to take action that may increase our contact with them. If we are distressed when around another person, we can choose to take action that results in a different emotional outcome.

Emotions are one part of ourselves only

Emotions are one part of ourselves—they are not the total of us. Other parts are our logical rational minds, our thinking selves, our creative selves, our physical selves, and our religious or spiritual selves.

Opening to emotions

For emotions to provide useful information about ourselves and our environment effectively we obviously have to be aware of our emotions in the first instance. In the past, we may have needed to keep our emotions away by burying or avoiding them. This may have enabled us to survive extremely difficult situations. Keeping emotions away can remain an effective skill to use in the future provided we use it sparingly and consciously, such as by choosing to distract ourselves. It is important, however, that we do this as little as possible, so that we can gradually begin to access the benefits of awareness of our emotions. Commitment to and practice of awareness of your emotions can significantly contribute to your recovery. Practice may include taking a moment or five minutes once or several times a day to reflect upon what you are feeling and putting a name to your emotion.

Recognizing emotions

♦ **Anger** is a stress response to real or perceived danger and causes a rush of adrenaline and increased blood flow to our muscles. Our muscles may tense up, especially in the shoulders and neck, as the body gets ready to fight or run (fight/flight response). We might be aware of clenched teeth, fist-making, or folded arms. Our heart and breathing may speed up and we may be thinking critical thoughts.

♦ **Fear** is also a stress response to real or perceived danger and also causes a rush of adrenaline, and we may experience some of the same body responses as with anger (tight muscles, rapid breathing). There may be an experience of dread and anxiety and an urge to get away. Thoughts may be worry type of thoughts.

♦ **Sadness** often occurs in response to a loss (recent or past) of something we value or valued. Sadness may be felt physically as a lump in the throat, a sense of heaviness, or a sense of emptiness. Energy may be low. Many people cry when they are sad. Thoughts may be negative, pessimistic, or focused on particular sad events.

♦ **Happiness** is more likely to occur when we are engaged in activities that are pleasurable (fun), purposeful, or meaningful, and when we are relaxed or remembering a positive experience. Happiness may be experienced as a sense of lightness, contentment, or fulfilment. We may be energetic, having a 'spring in our step'. We may feel peaceful and at one with the world. We may feel buoyant and confident. Thoughts may be positive, optimistic, and hopeful.

Primary and secondary emotions
(Linehan, 1993b)

This concept, described variously by Linehan, Ellis, and others, is really valuable and can greatly assist your recovery. If the description below is not clear enough to you, discuss the concept with your therapist.

A primary emotion is an emotion that we experience in response to an internal or external event. A secondary emotion is an emotion we can have about the primary emotion on the basis of our self-critical beliefs about the primary emotion.

For example, anxiety about attending a job interview is a primary feeling. If we then have a self-critical belief about our anxiety such as, 'I should not be anxious', then it is likely that we will have additional feelings such as more anxiety, guilt, shame, or sadness about the primary emotion of anxiety. We will now be anxious about being anxious or feel ashamed about being anxious or sad about being anxious. We can see how this will make the already challenging situation even harder. Not only do we have to deal with our primary anxiety we also have to deal with our secondary shame, guilt, sadness, or anxiety.

Secondary emotions are often more problematic than are primary emotions. This is because they are associated with self-critical self-beliefs, prevent us accessing our primary emotions, and confuse the picture when we are trying to identify our primary emotions.

The solution to the problem of secondary emotions is theoretically simple but challenging. The solution to getting rid of our secondary emotions is to be accepting of our primary emotions. This concept can have profound implications for your recovery. To be less distressed by our emotions, we need to be more welcoming and accepting of our primary emotions whatever they are. This includes not only emotions that are pleasurable but also those that are distressing, including sadness, anxiety, and anger. If we are able to do this, and act skilfully whatever our primary emotion, we are then left with our primary emotions only, without the additional burden of our secondary emotions. This can lift a great weight from our shoulders and our lives.

 Comment from Wendy

I tried avoiding feeling a lot of the time. When I then felt something like being angry, sad, or happy, I would give myself a hard time and feel guilty for feeling what I did. This made every emotion more distressing. Once I learned to be fully present in the moment, and accept how I felt, I was able to work on managing the primary emotion, and thereby gain some control of my emotional states.

Riding the wave

We conclude this section on emotions with 'Riding the Wave' written by colleagues of ours for one of their treatment groups.

Riding the Wave

One way of thinking about our emotions is to think of them like the ocean. If you imagine the sea, you might picture it as flat, calm and blue, or as crashing surf, or small rocking waves.

Just as the ocean can change, so can emotions. With the ocean, it is the weather that might cause changes—high winds or still sunny days can make a difference to how the waves react. In our lives, it can be problems with friends or family, stress about school, things that happen in our environment and around us that may affect our emotions.

Sometimes you can see a storm brewing that might whip the waves up, other times the change may happen with little warning. But what we know for certain, about the sea and about our emotions—they chop and change.

So, like waves, our emotions may at one moment be calm and serene, and at another rocky and angry. We might float along on a happy emotion, or be swept away by anger, we might experience small emotional ups and downs, or we might get dumped by a big wave of sadness and hopelessness.

We can either let our emotions push us around and move us along—or we can learn how to harness our emotions. We can learn to float with our feelings, letting them wash over us, or how to surf the big feelings, not letting them crash over us, but taking control, and riding the wave!

This group is about learning how to ride the waves of emotion—not to be swept away by them, but to recognize weather changes (emotional warning signs), go with the flow, and deal with getting wet. Once you know how to ride the waves, you should have the skills with you to surf any breaker that comes your way.

(Kindly printed with the permission of Kari Centre Riding the Wave DBT Programme.)

30

Is it what we do with emotions of anger, guilt, and regret that makes a difference?

→ Key points

- We do not necessarily have to act on our feelings and urges.

- We all feel anger at times. Anger may arise in response to feeling threatened or used.

- To be able to deal with our anger skilfully, we first have to identify that we are angry.

- Often the guilt we experience comes directly from our self-talk and the messages we were given as vulnerable children.

- Many people's lives have turned around when they were able to stop blaming themselves for damaging things others have done to them, such as sexual assault.

Anger

Most of us have experienced anger in a negative way at some time of our lives. Consequently, we may attempt to block and hide our own anger at all costs. Bottling up anger can lead to our anger smouldering and perhaps later exploding in ways that are ineffective or worse. We all feel anger at times. Anger may arise in response to feeling threatened or used. If this is the case, our anger can give us important information. The challenge is to be open to our angry feelings and also to have productive ways of dealing with our anger. There are ways to manage anger without taking it out inappropriately on other people or ourselves, or risking our health or safety.

In preparation for when you are next angry, you might want to reflect on the concept that we do not necessarily have to act on our feelings. If your anger is not constructive, ask yourself if you can make a commitment to try not acting on angry feelings immediately. That is, we can be angry and just notice the anger without acting upon the anger.

To be able to deal with our anger skilfully, we first have to identify that we are angry. Then we need to claim our anger as ours, 'I am angry', rather than 'You made me angry'. Other people don't make us angry, although we may appropriately become angry in response to something someone has said or done. Wherever possible, try to slow down and not act on your anger immediately unless it is essential for your safety that you do so.

What do you need to do about your angry feelings?

- Do you need to assert yourself?

- Do you need to alter or rectify a situation?

- Do you need to remove yourself from the situation?

- Do you need to talk with a friend or partner?

If you assess that assertively expressing your opinion to the person that you are angry with will be productive, helping you achieve your goals, then assertively and respectfully express your opinion using all of your interpersonal skills. On other occasions, your anger might guide you to rectify a situation without asserting yourself directly to any person.

If you assess that assertively expressing your opinion to the person that you are angry with will be harmful for you, perhaps because they are in positions of great power, then you might want to try venting the anger indirectly (e.g. talk to a friend/therapist, garden, housework). In these situations it will be really important to talk about this situation with your therapist.

Warning!

The information outlined assumes that you are not or will not be in danger of physical assault. If you are in a physically violent relationship or there is any danger of you being assaulted if you stand up for yourself, it is essential that you discuss how best to proceed with your therapist.

If anger is a problem for you, as soon as possible do a formal or informal chain analysis around your feeling angry. What were the predisposing vulnerabilities and prompting events? What were the ongoing links in the chain including your thoughts, emotions, and actions?

Some people have difficulty getting angry enough when circumstances are such that anger would be effective. This can lead to feelings of depression as we can end up being insufficiently assertive and even feel guilty that we are not giving or doing enough, or that the situation is our fault. In these circumstances, identifying and expressing your anger constructively can be most beneficial in your recovery.

On the other hand, excess anger can also understandably corrode (eat away)

 Comment from Wendy

I never used to let my angry feelings out, except by turning them upon myself. I was scared that if I started to let it out it would never stop. This assumption proved to be untrue. Now I attempt to deal with anger as it arises, trying to learn what my feelings are telling me and looking for ways to address the situation I am in.

our relationships. Excess anger can occur when there is too much anger being felt, too much anger expressed, or where angry criticisms are not balanced with large doses of validation and affirmation of the other person. As a general rule of thumb, for critical comments to have any chance of being heard by another person they need to be said in the ratio of 5–10 positive affirming and validating comments for each critical comment. Remember all human beings like being rewarded and dislike being told off. So, if anger is a strong feature for any of us and of any of our relationships, we will need actively to pursue how we are going to decrease this so that our anger does not corrode our relationship.

Guilt

If you feel guilty, it will be important for you first to explore whether you could have done anything different regarding what you are feeling guilty about and whether guilt is a reasonable response to the event/s. If guilt is justified then try do some repair and work at not repeating the behaviour in the future.

Often the guilt we experience comes directly from our self-talk and the messages we were given as vulnerable children or by people who did damaging things to us. Many of these messages are no longer true, if they ever were, and need to be re-examined.

If your guilt is about things that happened when you were a child or teenager, it is likely that you had little realistic capacity to have done anything different. It is very common for people who are victims of physical or sexual assault to blame themselves for what happened. If you were abused as a child by an adult, remember that adults are always the ones who need to take responsibility for the events, not the child. If you blame yourself for events of your childhood, we encourage you to discuss and explore this with your therapist. Many people's lives have turned around when they were able to stop blaming themselves for damaging things adults did to them as children such as sexual abuse. If you have been a victim of physical or sexual assault as an adult, remember that nobody has the right to assault people in this manner—this is entrenched in law in almost all countries.

If you have assessed self-compassionately that you have made a mistake or mistakes as an adult, then consider how you might be able to move forward. A small amount of guilt can sometimes be productive by motivating helpful and effective present or future behaviour. If your self-compassionate assessment is that that you erred in some way as an adult, establish whether you are feeling guilty over something that can be changed or over something that can't be changed. If there is something that you can constructively and effectively do to change or rectify the present or future, then do so.

On the other hand what has been done cannot be undone. Guilt will not undo what has been done. If guilt cannot influence our present and future behaviour then it serves no productive and helpful purpose. Punishing ourselves is not productive—neither we nor anybody else benefits. Guilt here serves only to keep us stuck and prevent our forward movement to recovery. It takes time to come to terms with our past mistakes, miss-steps, and the ways in which we have hurt others, as well as ourselves. It takes time to make peace with ourselves if we have had to live with the fall-out of traumatized lives.

Gentleness to ourselves and self-compassion will need to be cultivated. If this is difficult, discuss and explore with your therapist how you might try developing self-compassion and what the barriers might be to self-compassion.

The pathway to decreasing guilt in circumstances where we self-compassionately identify mistakes we made as adults is by acceptance—accepting what has happened and can't be changed. Acceptance in turn is assisted by making a commitment to learn from the past and doing our very best in the future. Trying one's best is an excellent strategy. It not only decreases guilt by enabling us to say to ourselves that we have tried the best that we could but also has the additional benefit of increasing the chances of successful recovery.

Regret

Regret may manifest with 'if-only's' that destructively play over and over in our minds; 'if only . . . didn't happen', 'if only I had a different childhood', 'if only I had learned . . . when I was younger'.

We all have some regrets about things that we would have liked to be different; however, regret can become problematical if it consistently absorbs our energies on things that can no longer be changed. When events happen that we don't like, it is completely understandable that we will struggle emotionally coming to terms with what has happened. It is understandable and normal to think, 'What if . . .' for a while.

Healing involves grieving and letting go of the 'if only's' and moving to something like, 'I would have liked . . ., however I can't change that, but I can now. . .'. In this position, regrets are lightly held, taking little energy. This frees up our energies for what can be changed. Successful grieving over past events leads to acceptance of what happened and recovery. Another pathway to healing is practising acceptance of what happened, which in turn can assist grieving and lead to recovery.

Problems arise if we do not complete this grieving over what has happened, keeping us stuck. If you feel stuck with regret or stuck grieving over past events, discuss with your therapist how you might be able to proceed to a pathway that will support your healing.

31

Is it what we do with impulsive urges that makes a difference?

➔ Key points

◆ The good news is that things don't just happen 'out of the blue'.

◆ By using methods to increase awareness, we can break situations down into miniscule parts and develop skills to control our impulses.

◆ Slow and steady is the way to practise controlling impulsive behaviours.

Changing from a Ferrari to a Morris Minor

With impulsivity, conscious decision-making, thought, and planning are limited or absent. When we act impulsively, it may just seem to happen 'out of the blue' without any lead up. The good news is that things don't just happen 'out of the blue'. By using methods to increase awareness, we can break situations down into miniscule parts and develop skills to control our impulses.

Increasing awareness is central to all the major therapies and can include attention control, mindfulness, chain analysis, and self-reflection practices. Whether you do a formal chain analysis or not, it will be important to identify predisposing factors and prompting events that have led to past impulsive action. Prompting events may be internal or external. Examples are criticism, being around certain people, or feeling rejected or blamed.

We then need to be alert in future situations to recognizing the prompting event as soon as possible. This will require practising self-reflection, awareness, and mindfulness.

Recognizing that we can have an urge to act and choose nevertheless not to act can be extremely helpful. Some people have referred to this as 'riding the urge'. DBT will have you note in a daily diary your urges, where applicable, to suicide, self-harm, substance use, gambling, unsafe sex, violence, binge eating, and other activities. 'Riding the urge' effectively prevents impulsive behaviour that we would later regret.

As stated before, it often feels like we move from the prompting event to the action with nothing in-between. The good news is that this is not the case. SAFE in Canada use the metaphor of a flame-lighter, fuse, and bomb. The prompting event lights the fuse, but we still have time to act (e.g. put out the fuse, remove ourselves from the situation) before the bomb explodes (the impulsive behaviour). With practice we can lengthen the fuse so that we have time to act and defuse the bomb so the impulsive behaviour is averted or minimized. Identifying an urge to act will indicate that the fuse has been lit. A slow process enables us to put into place the solutions that we will have brainstormed in earlier formal or informal chain analyses.

A colleague uses the analogy of a car (with the permission of Jane Barrington). For those of you not familiar with a Morris Minor, it was a basic car of the 1950s that was known for its slow acceleration in contrast say to a Ferrari known for its fast acceleration. If we are driving a Morris Minor, we have much more time to reflect before acting, than if we are driving a Ferrari. Behaving as though we are driving a Morris Minor allows us to rectify the situation before it is too late. Slow and steady is the way to practise controlling impulsive behaviours.

 Comment from Wendy

I used to firmly believe that my impulsive actions 'just happened'. Learning to slow the process down enabled me to put in place solutions and avert or minimize unwanted action. This gave me choices, a sense of power and helped me maintain healthier friendships.

32

Is it taking charge of our personal boundaries that makes a difference?

⊃ Key points

◆ Keys to healthy boundaries

   ◆ persuading ourselves about the need for boundaries;

   ◆ asserting with others the boundaries.

◆ Signs to evaluate our boundaries

   ◆ if we regularly lose our power when we are in relationships;

   ◆ if we regularly keep people away and feel lonely, isolated, and empty.

◆ Signs that our boundaries are about right

   ◆ when we feel sufficiently safe with and adequately connected to people.

What are personal boundaries?

Have you ever noticed how very little we speak to others when we are in a confined space such as a lift/elevator? This is probably because we are already physically closer to people than we would ideally like. Physically, we have crossed our and their ideal boundaries—we have entered each others' personal physical space.

Boundaries in this chapter refer to the *psychological space* we all have around us.

> ## Boundaries are the psychological space we have around us

Psychological boundaries are about choosing:

◆ what

◆ where

◆ how

◆ and with whom

we share and are open to others.

Interaction with others occurs at boundaries, ours and theirs. Examples include feeling comfortable in the presence of one person and uncomfortable in the presence of another person. This will be because we are comfortable or uncomfortable being psychologically close to the person.

Why have personal boundaries?

Boundaries ideally serve to allow us to control who we are open and intimate with and who we are close to or keep at a distance. Ideally our boundaries will open to allow in people that we want to know us and see us for who we are, thereby enabling closeness, connection, and intimacy. These people will be ones that we have evaluated as people we like, respect, and feel safe with. On the other hand, people we do not like or we evaluate as unsafe will be the ones with whom we want to have our boundaries up, so that they can't get close enough to us to use or hurt us.

As you may well be aware, this task is very challenging, especially if we have not had opportunities as children and adults to build up boundary successes. If we are in great need of connection, we might inappropriately open our boundaries, allowing people into our psychological space who are not deserving of our trust, who then hurt us. On the other hand, we might excessively and inappropriately put up our boundaries so that we do not allow people in who are safe, thereby depriving ourselves of healthy connection. A common situation for people with BPD is to fluctuate from one end to the other, allowing unsafe people in, and shutting safe people out. The challenge is to have a boundary that is flexible so that we can let people in when it is wise for us to do so and shut people out when it is wise for us to do so.

Boundary metaphors

Metaphors of boundaries that people have found useful to help with this concept include:

- zip or zipper able to be opened and closed as needed from the inside

- clam that opens and closes as needed from the inside

- castle wall with a drawbridge that is lowered and raised as needed from the inside

- building with window shutters that are opened or closed as needed from the inside.

These metaphors have a number of things in common

- All have a firm boundary

- That boundary is flexible and used as needed

- That boundary is controlled from inside.

It is critical that we, and not others, are in control of whether our boundaries are up or down. It is critical that we identify the mechanisms whereby we open up or close down, so that we can be in charge, wherever possible. This requires a mindfulness or awareness of ourselves and the world around us.

Healthy boundaries need to be

- Under our control

- Finely tuned

- Flexible (let in safe people, keep out unsafe people)

- Clear

- Assertive (not aggressive)

- Enable us to say 'yes' and 'no' when we want to.

Psychological boundaries

- Honour and respect ourselves

♦ Protect us

♦ Are a foundation for sound healthy relationships.

Healthy boundaries

♦ Allow intimacy

♦ Are not weapons to be used against people

♦ Are not invasive of others

> You walk caringly on my mat
> you behave respectfully in my house
> and the door will always be open
> The way you walk on the mats
> the way you behave in the house
> will determine whether or not the door and window will be opened
>
> Maori proverb translated by Ruth Tai—Printed with permission of Ruth Tai

Some characteristics of safe and unsafe people

Safe	Unsafe
Listen	Don't listen
Hear us	Don't hear us
Generally accepting of us	Generally rejecting of us
Non-judgemental	Judgemental
Real with us	False with us
Boundaries appropriate	Boundaries inappropriate
Boundaries clear	Boundaries unclear
Generally supportive	Generally competitive (want to beat us)
Generally reliable	Generally unreliable

(Charles L. Whitfield, MD, material from Boundaries and Relationships:
Knowing, Protecting and Enjoying the Self. Copyright 1993 by
Charles L Whitfield, MD. Adapted and reprinted with the permission
of Health Communications, Inc., www.hcibooks.com)

I am responsible for:	*Others are responsible for:*
My thoughts	Their thoughts
My behaviours	Their behaviours
My attitudes	Their attitudes
My values	Their values
My choices	Their choices
My limits	Their limits
My goals	Their goals
Expressing my talents	Expressing their talents
Taking charge of my life	Taking charge of their life

Healthy boundary		
Flexible	not	Rigid
Clear	not	Unclear

Personal boundaries survey

The following questions might help you explore whether your boundaries are healthy (present, clear, flexible, consistent) or unhealthy (absent, erratic, too open, too closed, too rigid, too loose).

I have difficulty saying 'no' to people

I feel as if my happiness depends on other people

I don't get close enough to people to be able to call on them at a time of need

I find myself getting involved with people who end up hurting me

I would rather attend to others than attend to myself

I am like a rock, people don't affect me

Others' opinions are more important than mine

People take or use things without asking me

I have difficulty asking for what I want or what I need

I lend people money and do not seem to get it back on time

Some people I lend money to don't ever pay me back

I would rather go along with another person than express what I'd really like to do

I spend my time and energy helping others so much that I neglect my own wants and needs

I find myself getting involved with people who end up being bad for me

I am shy, so people don't know what I am feeling or thinking

I tend to take on the moods of people close to me

I keep myself safe from people, but I get lonely

I have a hard time keeping a confidence

I tend to stay in relationships that are hurting me

I tend to get caught up in the middle of other people's problems

I tend to take on or feel what others are feeling

I put more into relationships than I get out of them

I keep a distance from people so that they can't reject me

I feel responsible for other people's feelings

My friends or acquaintances have a hard time keeping confidences which I tell them

(Charles L. Whitfield, MD, material from Boundaries and Relationships: Knowing, Protecting and Enjoying the Self. Copyright 1993 by Charles L. Whitfield MD. Adapted and reprinted with the permission of Health Communications, Inc., www.hcibooks.com)

Setting a healthy boundary

> **Warning!**
>
> **If you are in a physically violent relationship or there is any danger of you being assaulted if you stand up for yourself, it is essential that you discuss how best to proceed with your therapist. The information outlined on setting boundaries assumes that you are not or will not be in danger of physical assault.**

When we meet someone, we automatically set or don't set a boundary or a limit with them. If we have had negative boundary experiences or have trouble knowing what is 'right' for us, we need to make this a process that we deliberately and intentionally focus awareness on.

Those of us who are excessively wary of others may have boundaries that are too large and unable to be let down to let others in who could enrich our lives. In this situation, our therapy work might explore how we might be able to loosen up on our boundaries. For others who let people in too easily, therapy work may be about tightening up our boundaries.

We need to pay attention to what our emotions, thoughts, and bodies are telling us. Uncomfortable feelings or critical thoughts about another person may be cues that a boundary needs setting. Do you always feel like leaving the room, pulling away, or taking a step back when with a certain person? If we find ourselves thinking we do not like being around another person, it is time to reflect on whether we need to set a boundary, or change to one that suits the current state of affairs better.

Setting a healthy boundary is about doing what is right for ourselves. If we are not comfortable being in a room alone with someone, then a healthy boundary for us with that person might be being with them only in the company of others. If we feel comfortable shaking hands with someone, but not hugging them, then this might be a healthy boundary for us with that person.

An excellent strategy on meeting someone, who we want to shake hands with but not hug, is assertively to put our hand far out as we greet them, while holding the rest of our bodies well back. You might want to practise this with a friend. Sometimes people do not pick up on these non-verbal cues and we need to state clearly to them what is OK and what is not OK. We need to be clear and concise, without apology, and for most day to day situations assert ourselves calmly and preferably without anger. Achieving our objective will often be enhanced by assertively explaining the situation; however, we do not generally have to justify ourselves. You can offer a brief explanation if it feels right to do that. 'I prefer not to be touched' or 'I am not a touchy sort of person' are simple but clear statements that set a clear boundary.

Sometimes we will set a healthy boundary that is experienced as hurtful to the other person, even though that is not our intention. On these occasions it could well be that the relationship will be better for our clear healthy boundaries, even though setting these boundaries may be difficult for us. Healthy boundaries are a way to allow us to be comfortable and safe with those around us, and are a positive feature of relationships.

If we are not used to setting boundaries we may feel afraid of the other person's reaction, or embarrassed about stating our needs. This is not a reason not to do it, unless our actual safety would be jeopardized. If we do not tell another person where our boundary lies, they may not know they are psychologically or physically trespassing. Healthy people usually respect others who are clear about their boundaries. It takes a lot of the guessing and tip-toeing out of relationships. Healthy boundaries are good for all concerned.

When we set boundaries, we can often find the boundary being tested. We need to expect this; it is part of the human condition for people to check out whether we really mean what we say. We need then to politely remind the other person of the boundary and act in a manner that communicates to the other person that we mean it. The other person will only believe that our boundary is for real if we stick to the boundary consistently. After a few occasions of seeing us stick to our boundary, most people will back off, recognizing that we do in fact mean what we say. On the other hand, if we occasionally back down, we will find that people will recognize this and keep on with their previous behaviour.

Often the person who has the most trouble accepting our boundaries will be ourselves. Here, the key to healthy boundaries lies first with persuading ourselves of the need and only secondly persuading others that we have them.

33

Is it how we clarify our values and identity that makes a difference?

Key points

◆ Identify your most important values, roles, and energizing activities.

◆ Identify what gives you a sense of pleasure, fulfilment, meaning, and purpose.

◆ Focus on strengthening these areas of your life.

Who am I and what do I believe in? Clarifying values and identity

We might be a woman, man, mother, father, daughter, son, aunt, uncle, friend, employer, employee, PTA member, movie watcher, TV watcher, sports fan, left-of-centre voter, right-of-centre voter, food appreciator, music appreciator, singer, Scrabble player, walker, dancer, traveller, radio listener, weather watcher, bird watcher, news person, martial artist, wrestler, pacifist, environmentalist, religious person, spiritual person, agnostic, atheist, and any one of hundreds of other roles.

Within each of these roles there are differences too. Music appreciation may involve listening to or playing music. Listening to or playing music may involve, classic, instrumental, vocal, jazz, rock, folk, opera, etc. We might listen to music on the radio, from CDs, or attend a music club. If we play a musical instrument, this might be a guitar, cello, drum, piano, etc. If we are a singer we might sing by ourselves in the shower, hum a tune on the radio, belong to a music club or choir, or perform live.

Each of these roles carries different degrees of involvement. One person who likes Scrabble may play casually once every five years with a friend while another might play in competitions every week.

We might be outgoing, reflective, sociable, solitary, reclusive, gregarious, serious, funny, humorous, supportive, sensitive, insensitive, thin-skinned, thick-skinned, worry a lot, worry a little, get sad a lot, get happy a lot, organized, disorganized, express anger, bottle up anger, depend on others, or be self-reliant.

Exercises to clarify values and identity

Roles

You might want to write down one or two roles that you have. If you want, you might want to circle one or more from the list below:

....

....

....

....

woman	man	musician	reader	straight	gay
lesbian	daughter	son	brother	sister	mother
father	friend	employer	employee	movie person	TV person
sports fan	singer	walker	dancer	left-of-centre voter	right-of-centre voter

agnostic	food appreciator	radio listener	music appreciator	atheist	cook
weather watcher	news person	religious person	spiritual person	cleaner	cook

Values

From the following list, you might want to circle values that apply to you:

fun	money	friendship	family	integrity	energy
honesty	stimulation	structure	novelty	companionship	justice
creativity	compassion	success	humanity	caring	modern
traditional	autonomy	community	doing	being	change
acceptance	religion	spirituality	reliability	flexibility	firmness
fairness	kindness	artistic	organized	working	sport

You may want to write down your five core (or central) values:

....
....
....
....
....

Energizing

You might want to sit down quietly and brainstorm non-harmful things that energize you:

> ....
>
> ....
>
> ....
>
> ....

Focus on strengthening these areas of your life so that you have areas that you are skilled at and passionate about.

Pleasure

You might want to write down three or four non-harmful things that give you enjoyment:

> ....
>
> ....
>
> ....
>
> ....

Focus on strengthening these areas of your life so that you have areas of your life that generate pleasure.

Fulfilment, meaning, and purpose

You might want to sit down quietly and brainstorm three to four non-harmful things that you find fulfilling, meaningful, or purposeful:

> ....
>
> ....
>
> ....
>
> ....

Focus on strengthening these areas of your life.

 Comment from Wendy

I spent many years wondering who I was and what the meaning of my life was. I then discovered two areas in my life, especially, that I was and am good at and passionate about. I now put time and effort into these two areas.

One is my work. On enough days, I do make a small difference in someone's day. This gives me considerable pleasure and satisfaction.

The other is my role to my nieces and nephew as 'Aunty Wendy'. I try to be the very best 'Aunty Wendy' I can, and get a huge sense of satisfaction and self-worth from the effort I put into that role.

After many years of searching for who I was, I now feel I have a place in the world fulfilling these and other roles.

34

Is it how we relate to ourselves that makes a difference?

> **Key points**
>
> ◆ We all have value.
>
> ◆ We all have a right to be here.
>
> ◆ We need to find ways of recognizing and acknowledging our successes, achievements, and positive qualities, however small.
>
> ◆ Our favourite way of working towards improved self-esteem is via the pathway of acceptance of who we are at any single moment.
>
> ◆ We need to try be compassionate with ourselves, recognizing that we are doing the best that we know how—nobody we have met has said, 'I am going to get up today and deliberately make some poor decisions!'

Self-compassion

We need to explore how we can develop a way of relating to ourselves with compassion. This may be recognizing that we are managing as anybody else might do in the same circumstances or, where this is not accurate, that we are doing the best that we know how given our biological temperament and our past and current circumstances. This will make it a little easier to deal with the challenges of day to day life. Discuss with your therapist how you can build compassionate ways of relating to yourself and any barriers that you might have to self-compassion such as a belief that you do not deserve self-compassion.

> **We all have value**
>
> **We all have a right to be here**

 Comment from Wendy

I was, and still am to some extent very hard on myself—I expected nothing less than perfection, and anything a fraction short of perfection was a failure—another of my many failures. Over time I have learnt that like every other human, there are some things I am better at than others, and I was not going to be perfect at everything I do and every interaction I have with someone. Learning to accept that I am OK, even if I am not perfect has been a big learning curve with great rewards. I am much more casual now about minor things, 'not sweating the small stuff'. With important activities, while I still strive to do my very best, I am much more accepting if things don't work out. After all, how could I ask myself to do any more than my best? I am much kinder now towards myself, which helps me go about my world with a lightness I never had before.

Self-esteem

Spotlighting successes

We need to create an environment where our self-esteem can grow strong by identifying when we are putting ourselves down and finding alternative more effective ways of relating to ourselves. We need to find ways of recognizing and acknowledging our successes, achievements, and positive qualities, however small. We are not glibly suggesting that you 'Just be positive', which is almost always not helpful. If we could 'just be positive' we would have done so long ago. What we are suggesting though is to focus our attention on small positive qualities and small successes—a bit like a spotlight focusing on what we want to focus on. We need to be alert to self-talk that throws the spotlight on the negatives such as after a small success saying 'It was just a one off', or 'It won't last'. With a spotlight we are not discounting negatives but bringing positives into the light so that they can be seen, perhaps for the first time.

Self-esteem and success

Success and self-esteem have a circular relationship (Fig. 34.1).

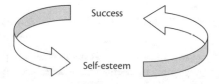

Having success and recognizing it (even small successes) increases our self-esteem. In turn, increased self-esteem supports us to venture forth wisely trying things, thereby opening up possibilities of more small successes. In fact, deliberately aiming for small successes is usually more important than aiming for large successes as it increases our chances of building successes and consequent self-esteem. Explore with your therapist how you might plan a sequence of activities starting with the smallest activity that is likely to be successful, progressing to larger activities once you have built up some successes.

When we venture forward we will not get everything right—we will not be effective at everything. The journey of moving forward usually involves aiming to be effective more often than not, accepting times of not getting it right as part of the journey. If we never venture forward due to our desire not to fail, we might miss, say, 20 opportunities. We may not have failed at anything but we have deprived ourselves of 20 opportunities of success. Depending on the nature of the activities, it is likely that our lives will be better off if we venture forth despite our anxiety about failure and find that we fail three times and succeed 17 times.

Comment from Wendy

At my worst, I lay in bed all day. There was no way that I was going to recover doing that. A small initial success was getting out of bed and walking to the shops. My self-esteem improved again when I moved into a household that expected me to contribute by being responsible for the weekly food shopping and my share of the cleaning. Later a large success was a part-time voluntary job as a teacher's aide that filled my days with purpose and, later still, paid employment. These initially small and later large successes promoted my independence, recovery, and self-esteem.

Self-acceptance

Except for uncommon situations the following are our thoughts on self-acceptance.

Our favourite way of working towards improved self-esteem is via the pathway of acceptance of who we are at any single moment. This is a very compassionate way of relating to ourselves. Accepting ourselves in the moment is not passive resignation and does not preclude changing our behaviour in the future. When we enter therapy after all, we do so because we want to change our behaviours. It is just saying to ourselves that we are doing as well as we can, given our biology (genes), past and current circumstances, and, where applicable, that we want to do better. This is a central assumption in DBT. Nobody that we have met has said 'I am going to get up today and deliberately make some poor decisions that will make life worse for me'.

Self-acceptance is often a treatment goal. Explore with your therapist ways of working towards this.

35

Is it how we relate to others that makes a difference?

> **→ Key points**
>
> ◆ As you heal and develop awareness of yourself and the world around you, you will be able to influence your relationships becoming more effective.
>
> ◆ Relationships tend to work best when we come together from positions of clarity about who we are and what we want.
>
> ◆ The desired levels of connection will vary over time and with different people.
>
> ◆ Starting relationships slowly is generally wise.
>
> ◆ People are more likely to be genuinely generous with us if we express our needs in an assertive but not demanding way.
>
> ◆ Try not to take natural progressions personally—they are a fact of life.

Most human beings are drawn to some level of relationship and human connection. However, many people with BPD find relationships difficult, and 'unstable relationships' is one of the DSM-IV diagnostic criteria for BPD. Difficulties in relationships may include fears of rejection, being left, let down, getting hurt, hurting others, getting used, getting abused, getting disappointed, being vulnerable, losing identity, being used as a doormat, and fears of not being able to manage without the other person.

There is hope. As you heal and develop awareness of yourself and the world around you, you will be able to influence your relationships, increasing the likelihood of more effective relationships.

Values, identity, and relationships

Some of us may feel that we don't really know who we are, and fear losing what little we do know about who we are, if we get close to someone—we may fear losing ourselves. Others of us who don't really know who we are may want to get close to another person so as to take on the other person's identity and values. What is important in moving forward in both these situations is to increase our awareness of who we are by clarifying our values, beliefs, likes, and dislikes. This leaves us better placed to enter a relationship on more solid ground. Relationships tend to work best when we come together from positions of clarity about who we are and what we want. In this situation, neither party loses who they are as intimacy develops. Healthy intimacy is enhanced by coming into relationships from a solid knowing of who we are.

Connection

In our relationships, we need to aim for connection that is just right—neither too close nor too far away. Too far and we may feel lonely and isolated, too close and we may feel engulfed. Many of us have considerable difficulty getting this balance right, and may alternate between pulling people towards us and pushing them away. Take some time to reflect on the level of closeness that would be desirable for you in your different relationships. Draw on your past relationships to guide you here and discuss this issue with your therapist. Desirable levels of connection will vary over time and with different people. For example, the level of closeness will obviously be greater with a friend than with an acquaintance.

Start slowly

Starting relationships slowly is generally wise. This slow pace enables us to tame our impulsivity and provides the necessary time to assess wisely whether the person is deserving of our trust. Time also supports our reconciling the likable and less likable aspects of the person and the relationship. Most sexual relationships and many other intense relationships start with a 'honeymoon' period, during which time we are vulnerable to making decisions that might not be in our best interests. Of course, we need not to be so slow that we never enter into any relationships.

Communication

We may wish people would understand our needs more, not realizing that for someone to understand our needs we need to explain to them in a respectfully assertive non-confrontational way what our needs are. People are more likely to be genuinely generous with us if we express our needs in an assertive but not demanding way.

While a person's facial expression and body posture are clues, nobody can observe someone else's emotions. If it is important enough, we may need to ask the person what they are feeling. If we do not, we run the risk of getting it wrong. For the same reasons, if we want to be sure that the other person knows what we are feeling, we will need to tell them.

Emotions connect us and if we struggle with intense unstable emotions it is understandable that we may have difficulty in our relationships with others. The emotion that lies behind our words may make our communication too weak or too strong. Sometimes our body language or facial expression does not match what our words are saying, so we send out a mixed message. If we fear rejection, we may be too timid and unassertive. If we fear being controlled or we are intensely angry, we may be overly assertive— aggressive. Learning when and how to express our emotions is an important skill in making and maintaining relationships. Learning effective ways of making our needs known, and making requests of others are essential skills when building relationships.

Personalizing

Personalizing is an ineffective way of thinking where we give ourselves a hard time by assuming without enough evidence that we are to blame for events that are not under our control. An example is blaming ourselves if a partner drinks, gambles, or is violent. Difficult as it can be to accept, therapists leave jobs or go on maternity leave and friends move town, etc. Where these moves are unrelated to ourselves, we need to try not take these natural progressions personally—they are a fact of life, and would have happened whether or not we were a part of that person's life.

DBT interpersonal effectiveness skills (Linehan, 1993b)

DBT encourages us to prioritize whether achieving our objective, keeping the relationship or our self-esteem is the most important in any interpersonal situation, and act accordingly. Of course, one can sometimes attend to all these at the same time also. DBT has acronyms that highlight key points for interpersonal effectiveness.

When focusing on the objective, the acronym 'DEARMAN' stands for;

describe the situation

express your feelings and opinions

assert yourself

reinforce the person ahead of time

be **m**indful of objectives

appear confident

negotiate alternative solutions.

When focusing on the relationship, the acronym 'GIVE' stands for;

gentle

interested

validate the other person's feelings and opinions

easy manner.

When focusing on our self-esteem, the acronym 'FAST' stands for;

fair to ourselves

not overly **a**pologetic behaviour

stick to our values

truthful.

Linehan (1993b; printed with the permission of Guilford Press)

Liking to disliking and back again

Kreisman and Straus (1991), *I hate you, don't leave me*, use the term that sums up the dilemma we may feel in our relationships. We may see people as 'all good' or 'all bad', and find it difficult accepting that we all have more and less likable parts. When we see people as 'all good' or 'all bad', we will swing on a pendulum in the relationship. One day the person is everything we want them to be—kind, caring, fun, etc., and we elevate them onto an inappropriately ideal 'pedestal'. The trouble with pedestals is that people will eventually fall off. The next day when the person is not at their best (or worse) we suddenly push them off the pedestal that we put them on in the first place and they become, in our eyes, a dreadful person. It is easy to see the devastating effects this can have on ourselves and our relationships.

When we learn to accept that each person is made up of a combination of qualities we like and like less, it is easier not to personalize the person's being off colour that day as our fault, and instead 'ride the wave', knowing that the aspects of the person we care about are still there, and will manifest again.

Liking to disliking our therapist and back again

Consider whether you are elevating your therapist onto an idealized pedestal and whether you may want to discuss this with your therapist. If you find your views of your therapist changing suddenly so that you think that they are dreadful, you are likely to have a strong urge to fire them. Unless your therapist is engaging in professionally unethical behaviour (physical/verbal abuse, sexual contact, or other behaviours), we strongly encourage you to recognize that this is a common feeling that people with BPD have and make a commitment to staying in therapy long enough to be able to discuss your feelings and thoughts thoroughly with your therapist. We really mean it when we say that relationship difficulties with your therapist can be wonderful opportunities for assertion, self-awareness, relationship repair, and managing conflict, if well processed.

If you have a thought that your therapist has not understood you, try recognizing this for what it is—a thought. That is, it might be fact or it might not be fact. All you can be sure of is that you have a thought that they do not understand you. You can explore whether your thought is an accurate representation by being open and telling them what you are thinking and asking for their response.

We are not saying that all problems that you experience in your relationship with your therapist are your problems or can be talked out. However, what have you got to lose by staying long enough to see whether you can talk out the problems? The worst that can happen is that you spend a few more sessions discussing these issues. If you are not in therapy, you cannot benefit from therapy!

Success of therapy may hinge on how you and your therapist manage these conflicts with each other.

The same principles can be applied to other relationships where we find ourselves in sudden shifts between liking and disliking others.

Reflect before permanently rejecting others

Synthesizing our mixed feelings for others will go a long way to avoiding ending relationships unnecessarily during a period of dissatisfaction with the other person.

Another way of avoiding ending relationships unnecessarily is to be mindful of the role of rejection in our lives. For some of us, if we feel we are about to be rejected or abandoned we may leave the relationship first, without ever knowing what the other person was thinking or feeling. If our perceptions are not checked out we could tragically end relationships unnecessarily.

These principles apply to our relationships with therapist, friends, and family.

On the other hand, avoid staying in harmful relationships

In our important relationships it is important for us to be safe from physical, sexual, and verbal abuse. To do this we need to have reasonable self-awareness, especially of our boundaries, and also an awareness of the characteristics of the other person.

If the network of people in our lives is fairly small, we may hang on to a relationship at all costs, even if the relationship is harmful. Human beings are powerfully drawn to being in a relationship and to human connection. This can sometimes be so strong that we might end up staying in relationships despite the relationships being harmful for us.

Another reason for staying in unhealthy relationships involves being drawn to somebody who we see as strong and powerful to counterbalance our feelings of weakness or powerlessness, and the person has an unhealthy power over us in a manner that is harmful or even abusive.

Repair

The intense feelings and anger we may feel can often lead to damaged relationships or to being estranged (not speaking or on bad terms) from people we really care about. On other occasions, damage to relationships may have occurred if we asked more of people than they could sustain. As you increase your awareness of yourself and others, gain more control of your emotions, begin to see people as 'wholes', instead of 'all good' or 'all bad', and begin to develop boundaries and self-worth, you may decide to try building bridges with some of the people where relationships have been damaged.

If you do, here are some tips.

- Use non-judgemental 'I' statements that describe observable facts. This can include your feelings. For example, 'When you said ..., I felt hurt' rather than 'You hurt me when...'.

- Avoid inflammatory words such as 'You bastard'.

- Apologize for any hurt you may have caused the other person, if accurate.

- Explain that you may have been wrong or perceived something incorrectly, if accurate.

- Tell the person that you value them and would like to mend the relationship.

- Explain that you are working on your issues trying to improve your behaviours.

- Ask them what behaviours they would need to see from you for them to consider repair.

This obviously won't always work, but it has a better chance than not trying at all.

 Comment from Wendy

My behaviour resulted eventually in my family not feeling able to have anything to do with me. I was not invited to and did not attend my brother's and sister's weddings.

After many years of not speaking, repair began to take place, precipitated by my mother's terminal illness. I finally met my brother-in-law, sister-in-law, and niece for the first time.

My mother and I talked through many events that had caused friction, at least in my mind, between us over the years. Many of the events where I had felt slighted, overlooked, and even emotionally abused were so different in her memory. She had seen me as an extremely sensitive child and had felt she lacked the skills to deal with such a challenging child, so dealt with me the best she knew how. Many of the hurts that had festered inside me for years as signs of my inadequacy were so insignificant to her that she could not recall them, even with prompting.

Mum and I spent many hours talking over several months, and I eventually, and for the first time, felt comfortable in the knowledge that she loved me as much as my brother and sister. I felt a wound healing—my relationship with my mother was repaired. Definitely late, but definitely not too late.

I also gradually repaired my relationships with other family members and am delighted now to be 'Aunty Wendy' to my wonderful nieces and nephew.

Of all the joys of recovery, my close relationship with my family has to be one of the greatest.

36

Is it how we create pleasure that makes a difference?

Key points

♦ While it makes obvious sense that having pleasure can be extremely helpful towards recovery, this is not always easy to do.

♦ You might need to try many activities, some of them a few times, before you discover those that give you pleasure. In this way you can build a collection of suitable activities.

While it makes obvious sense that having pleasure can be extremely helpful towards recovery, this is not always easy to do. The following is a list of reasons why having pleasure can be difficult to achieve:

♦ You may have had so little pleasure in your life that you are just not that knowledgeable about what you find pleasurable.

♦ You may, like many people with BPD, believe that you do not deserve pleasure.

♦ You may believe that it is OK to have pleasure, but find it difficult to nurture yourself.

♦ You may believe that you deserve pleasure but that others should provide this for you, rather than you having to go out and make it happen yourself.

♦ You may believe that you deserve pleasure and know what pleases you, but find it hard getting into the mood to do pleasurable activities.

If any of these situations apply to you, it will be important that you discuss this with your therapist so that you can begin to find ways of assisting your recovery via having more pleasurable experiences.

Many therapists will have a list or lists of pleasurable activities that you might be able to engage in. We have supplied a small list just to get you started, after which you can make a list of your own. The challenge then will be to schedule a time to do the activity and in due course regular times to do a number of the activities. In the early stages we are aiming just to have a small amount of pleasure for a small amount of time. Of course, if you experience large amounts of pleasure for large amounts of time that will be great. However, start with realistic expectations. Better to start small and build successful pleasurable experiences than start large and be disappointed. You might need to try many activities, some of them a few times, before you discover those that give you pleasure. In this way you can build a collection of suitable activities. The only rule is that the pleasurable activity will not be harmful to you or anyone else.

Our starting list is obviously not comprehensive but intended to stimulate you to develop your own list:

♦ Sitting in the sun	♦ Shopping
♦ Watching a good movie	♦ Window shopping
♦ Walking in the fresh air	♦ Cooking
♦ Watching the stars	♦ Eating tasty food
♦ Looking at plants	♦ Listening to music
♦ Watching birds flying	♦ Reading a book
♦ Making a scrapbook	♦ Watching the news on TV
♦ Drawing	♦ Listening to radio (music, current affairs, talk-back)

- ◆ Painting
- ◆ Watching sport
- ◆ Playing sport
- ◆ Playing cards with others
- ◆ Playing cards by ourselves
- ◆ Playing computer games
- ◆ Surfing interesting sites on the internet

- ◆ Visiting a friend/family
- ◆ Having a dinner party
- ◆ Having a bath with oils
- ◆ Having a massage
- ◆ Stroking the cat or dog
- ◆ Giving and receiving a hug

My list of pleasurable activities I will consider doing:

....
....
....
....

....
....
....
....

....
....
....
....

....
....
....
....

....
....
....
....

....
....
....
....

....
....
....
....

37

Is it how we deal with 'flashbacks' that makes a difference?

> **⊃ Key points**
>
> ◆ Flashbacks refer to distressing intrusive experiences that may be thoughts, emotions, or perceptions (sounds, visions, smells, tastes, or body sensations) that are the same or similar to past unpleasant or traumatic experiences. The experiences may quickly 'flash us back' (flashback) to the past, so to speak.
>
> ◆ It will be helpful to identify the prompting events and chain of events that lead to flashbacks and then work on changing events in the chain to reduce flashbacks occurring.
>
> ◆ During the flashback tell yourself that you are not going mad, get yourself 'grounded', and re-establish your awareness of being in the present.

What are 'flashbacks'?

Flashbacks refer to distressing intrusive experiences that may be thoughts, emotions, or perceptions (sounds, visions, smells, tastes, or body sensations) that are the same or similar to past unpleasant or traumatic experiences. The experiences may quickly 'flash us back' (flashback) to the past, so to speak. Common perceptions are images and sounds, but also taste, smell, and body sensations. Common emotions are feeling trapped, powerlessness, fear, and dread.

Flashbacks can be extremely frightening and confusing experiences. Not only are the emotions and body sensations frightening *per se*, but they can also be additionally frightening as they often do not appear understandable as they may not appear to be related to present reality. This confusion can then generate increased fear, including the fear of 'going mad'.

Flashbacks often bring back emotions from past trauma. As the flashback happens, it is as if we become as we were at the time of the trauma, forgetting that we have our current self available for comfort, protection, and grounding. If the trauma occurred when we were a child, we might have experiences of being the 'child'; we were forgetting that we have our current 'adult' selves available for comfort, protection, and grounding.

For some people flashbacks seem to come out of the blue for no apparent reason. The very fact that flashbacks may seem to be unpredictable might leave us feeling that flashbacks are uncontrollable and that stopping flashbacks is impossible.

What we can do?

There are three areas for us to explore taking charge, each suited for use at different times.

Understanding the prompting events and chain of events

It will be helpful to identify the prompting events and chain of events that lead to flashbacks by self-reflection, chain analysis, and attention control/mindfulness. As discussed in Chapter 26, this process can enable us to take charge and understand the sequence of events, changing flashbacks from something that is unpredictable that seems to come out of the blue to an experience that while distressing is understandable and predictable. Sometimes we can identify prompting events that make sense in that they are reminders of past trauma.

Once we can identify the chain of events that lead to flashbacks, we can then explore solutions that will decrease the frequency and/or intensity of future flashbacks. Of course when we understand these sequences, we will know that we are not 'going mad', which will decrease our anxiety.

During the flashback

Tell yourself that you are having a flashback.

If you can, try telling yourself that it is JUST a flashback. This is not to minimize the reality or severity of your distress but to try to decrease some of the additional fears, such as fears of 'going mad'. This can then have the effect of decreasing distress.

You might find it helpful to tell yourself that you are not 'going mad' if this is a concern of yours.

Remind yourself that the worst is over. The feelings and sensations you are experiencing are likely to be your body and mind's *memories* of the past.

'Get grounded'. 'Getting grounded' is a metaphor to describe a return to a psychological solid base. A psychological solid base is usually awareness of something that is familiar, certain, and predictable. Get grounded in whatever way works best for you. For some people this means focusing attention on their breathing, for others their feet on the floor and body on the chair, and for others walking around their home noting familiar sights. Some people stamp their feet on the ground.

If you are planning to focus on your breathing, ensure that you practise breathing in a manner that decreases rather than increases your anxiety levels. If you are not familiar with this distinction or how to breathe effectively at times of stress, discuss this with your therapist.

Re-establish to the present. Begin to use your senses in the present. Look around and see the colours in the room, the shapes of things, the people near, etc. Listen to the sounds in the room; your breathing, traffic, birds, people, cars, etc. Feel your body and what is touching it; your clothes, your own arms and hands, the chair or floor supporting you.

Take time after the flashback has passed to tend to yourself compassionately.

Late in recovery

Until now we have talked about flashbacks as a problem to be avoided and an experience to be got out of as soon as possible. Occasionally, late in your recovery when your life has well and truly stabilized, you might explore with your therapist the concept of deliberately bringing on some of the experiences previously described as flashbacks. The idea of deliberately trying to generate some of these experiences is to stay successfully with the experiences until the distressing feelings subside, making the memories of the past less powerfully intrusive in your current life. It is definitely not necessary that you deliberately bring on these flashback type of experiences to recover, but for some people it may be helpful to solidify changes that you have made.

> **Be patient. It takes time to learn ways of coping in the here and now. It takes time to heal the past. Take good care of yourself.**

38

Is it how we deal with crises that makes a difference?

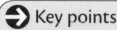 Key points

- It is critical that you do whatever you can to keep yourself safe.

- When a crisis occurs you will obviously try your best to put in place any or all of your learning from your therapy and from having read this book.

- For distracting activities to be effective they need to be compelling enough to draw our attention to them and away from the problem.

- BPD is a condition where crises exist whether we like it or not. Crises are a central part of the condition but do not have to be a central part of your life as you recover. Once you are beyond the worst of crises you will probably no longer have the condition called BPD.

Keeping yourself safe

In crises you will be more vulnerable to behaviours that decrease your safety including, for example, severe numbing out (dissociating) and urges to suicide, self-harm, use substances. It is critical that you do whatever you can to keep yourself safe.

Preparing for crises

Preparing for crisis situations will be very important and has been covered under that heading in Section 2 and also in several chapters in Section 3 (awareness, thinking, doing, feeling, impulsivity, boundaries, identity and values, relationships, physical health, flashbacks, pleasure).

Map for surviving crises

Linehan (2003) describes three healthy responses to painful problems ('Solve the problem, change how you feel, accept it'), which we have teased out in the box below.

---

1. Identify the problem.

2. Ask yourself if you can solve the problem.

3. If you can solve the problem, solve it.

4. If you can't solve the problem, ask yourself how you can try feeling better about the problem.

5. Try feeling better about the problem.

6. If you can't solve the problem and can't feel better about the problem, try feeling better in other ways.

7. If none of this works, try accepting things just as they are without making things worse.

When a prompting event occurs and you are aware your emotional barometer is rising excessively, STOP. If you have a written plan, find it and read it slowly. Is it possible to problem solve and ease the problem? If not, is there something that you can do to make yourself feel better? If not, can you try just accepting things as they are for the time being?

In some situations we cannot solve the problem, cannot make ourselves feel better about the problem, and cannot make ourselves feel better in other ways. When this occurs there are few options left but to accept the present moment, sit it out, and not make things worse. Distress does wax and wane.

When a crisis occurs you will obviously try your best to put in place any or all of your learning from your therapy and from having read this book. As such the following list on what to do in a crisis is a brief summary of key aspects of Section 3 of this book.

When you are aware of a crisis arising

◆ Identify the problem.

◆ If you can solve the problem do so, if you can't solve the problem try to feel better about the situation, if you can't do either try acceptance (Linehan, 1993b).

◆ Remember your crisis planning.

◆ Find your written plan and read it.

◆ Invite self-awareness by self-reflection, chain analysis of events, or mindfulness.

◆ Reflect whether your thinking is effective or ineffective (JCOB: jumping to conclusions, catastrophizing, overgeneralizing, black and white thinking).

◆ Ask yourself whether your emotions are primary or secondary (where you are giving yourself a hard time unnecessarily) and if secondary try letting them go.

◆ Ask yourself if you can try just accepting your primary emotions.

◆ Stop and ask whether you are moving too fast and adjust accordingly.

◆ Ask yourself whether your boundaries are healthy and adjust accordingly.

◆ Ask yourself if you want to accept your urges without acting on them.

◆ Ask yourself whether you want to try nurture yourself with pleasing activities.

◆ Ask yourself if you want to try a distraction activity.

◆ Ask yourself if you are being compassionate to yourself.

Distraction and pleasing activities

Distraction is a way of avoiding a problem. If we always used distraction, we would never solve problems or develop the skills to solve problems. It would be an ineffective method of going through life. However, distraction can be useful to help us get through a situation that we can't solve, without causing further deterioration in that situation. Although distraction might seem to be an overly simplistic solution to distress resulting from complex problems, it has been shown to be one of the more effective ways human beings make themselves feel better when they can't solve the problem.

Many distraction activities will be pleasurable while others will be pure distraction. For example, intense exercise may not be that pleasing for some, but can be very distracting. Holding ice blocks safely instead of self-harming is unlikely to be pleasing, but can be very distracting. On the other hand, watching compelling movies or listening to favourite music might be both distracting and pleasing.

One of the strengths of doing pleasing activities by ourselves is that we do not have to rely on others being around to 'pick us up', although we might choose to call someone or spend time with someone as one of our tools.

For distracting activities to be effective they need to be compelling enough to draw our attention to them and away from the problem. We may need to try more than one activity before finding one that works. Sometimes an activity that worked one day will not be effective the next and we will need to try another activity. Some people save up a particularly effective distraction strategy for those times when it is really needed, thereby making the most of the distracting effect of novelty. Other people find that the more familiar a distracting activity is the more grounding and settling it is, so actually practise using the activity frequently.

Our list of distracting and pleasing activities will be very individualized. Some people enjoy having a bath or going for a walk while others do not.

Please refer to the list of pleasing activities in Chapter 36 that you can use both at usual times and at times of crises.

The following is a list of additional activities that we have included here because we thought they might be quite compelling and therefore be of value as distraction activities for some people. The list is not comprehensive but rather intended to stimulate you to make your own list afterwards.

◆ Vigorous exercise subject to appropriate fitness levels	◆ Massage cream and oils into your skin yourself
◆ Computer games	◆ Wrap face in a very warm damp facecloth
◆ Puzzles and crosswords	◆ Swim
◆ Baking	◆ Sing loudly

- Perfume oils

- Holding ice safely in hand

- Eating hotly spiced food

- Eating any heavily spiced food

- Eating a slice of lemon

- Chewing fresh gum

- Chewing strong peppermints

- Having a 'hot as you can safely cope with' bath

- Having a 'hot as you can safely cope with' shower

- Having a 'long as you can' shower

- Having a safe massage from someone else

- Brush hair safely

- Any hobby that is engaging and keeps you busy:
  - crocheting
  - reading
  - sketching
  - painting
  - playing a musical instrument
  - writing poetry
  - needle-point
  - wood-working
  - leather-crafts, etc.

My list of safe distracting activities I will experiment with:

....
....
....
....

....
....
....
....

....
....
....
....

....
....
....
....

```
......................................................................................
......................................................................................
......................................................................................
......................................................................................
......................................................................................
......................................................................................
......................................................................................
......................................................................................
......................................................................................
......................................................................................
......................................................................................
......................................................................................
```

This chapter on dealing with crises brings together much of our learning on recovery. BPD is a condition where crises exist whether we like it or not. Crises are a central part of the condition but do not have to be a central part of your lives as you recover. Once you are beyond the worst of crises you will no longer have the condition called BPD.

 Comment from Wendy

I never wanted to prepare for crises—surely every crisis would be the last. It was hard for me to accept that learning to manage crises was an important part of my recovery—to me that was like accepting that crises were OK. And guess what?—I now know that difficult times happen to all of us and what we all require is simply to have the skills to get through the difficult times.

Although reluctant, I was persuaded to develop a written plan to deal with crises, which sat in my drawer unused for a very long time. One day, in yet another crisis, I decided I wanted to do something differently—I was totally sick of the crisis routine—so I looked at the plan and did some things in it—with some success. While it took some while for the frequency and intensity of crises to decrease reliably, by accepting crises would occur and having strategies to manage them, I eventually learnt to deal better with distressing times.

39

Is it how we manage our physical health that makes a difference?

➡ Key points

- As our physical condition impacts on our emotional well-being, it is worth attending to, not only for its direct physical benefits but also for the beneficial effects on our emotional state.

- It is important that we sleep as well as possible to support our resilience (hardiness) in dealing with our day to day tasks.

- We need to eat a regular balanced nutritious diet to give our bodies the fuel it needs to keep going, especially at difficult times.

- One of the hypotheses why exercise helps with depression is that exercise stimulates the release of our own 'feel good' chemicals called endorphins.

- Alcohol and other non-prescribed mind altering drugs cloud our minds and can mess with our bodies.

As our physical condition impacts on our emotional well-being, it is worth attending to, not only for its direct benefits but also for the beneficial effects on our emotional state.

Sleep

Many people have sleep problems. Our experience is that this is particularly common and important for people with BPD. It is important that we sleep as well as possible to support our resilience (hardiness) in dealing with our day to day tasks. If you have sleep difficulties, discuss this with your therapist. Some of the basic principles that you and your therapist might explore are:

♦ Establish a suitable regular time of going to sleep.

♦ Establish a suitable regular time of waking and getting out of bed.

♦ Do not sleep-in beyond your suitable regular time of waking. Even though it is tempting to sleep-in if we have had a poor nights sleep, this can really disturb our sleep rhythms. So save sleeping-in for critical and unusual times only.

♦ Do not sleep in the day.

♦ If you can't fall asleep within 20 minutes, get up and do something exceptionally unsatisfying until you feel sleepy. The idea here is to not 'reward' yourself in any way for being awake. If this strategy is not effective over time try instead just to lie as still as you can, thereby receiving as little physical stimulation as possible.

♦ Do not vigorously exercise for at least 4 hours before bedtime.

♦ Develop regular sleep rituals. These prepare our bodies for sleep.

♦ Only use bed for sleeping—so that going to bed tells your body it is sleep time.

♦ Gradually cut back on caffeine (coffee, tea, cola drinks) as much as possible especially in the afternoon and evening. Caffeine is a stimulant.

♦ In the 2–3 hours before sleep, engage in activities that are slowing or relaxing and avoid activities that are too stimulating or worrying.

♦ If worry is a problem, develop strategies with your therapist for this.

♦ Make sure your bed is comfortable.

♦ Do what you can so that your bedroom is quiet and comfortable.

♦ Do what you can to make your bedroom dark. Sleep is triggered by darkness.

Eating

Food is fuel. Many of us forget this. If we do not put fuel into a car we won't be surprised when it stops going. If we do not eat a regular balanced nutritious diet we will deprive our bodies of the fuel our bodies need to keep going, especially at difficult times. People with BPD usually have enough difficulties, without exacerbating things by inadequate nutrition. Excessive deprivation of calories makes us all feel miserable—so miserable that we cannot possibly sustain this situation and we then may overeat. Yo-yo dieting (feast and famine) will make it really hard for us to deal with day to day struggles. The goal is to find a way of eating that is sustainable for the rest of our lives.

If any of the following apply to you, it is important that you discuss them with your therapist:

◆ Deliberately vomiting after eating

◆ Using laxatives or purgatives

◆ Binge eating

◆ Others telling you that you are too thin

◆ Dieting

◆ Concern about your body shape

◆ Concern about your weight

◆ Body mass index (BMI) of 20 or less (World Health Organization definition of underweight has a BMI of 20 or less)

To work out your BMI you can use the following equation

$$\frac{Weight(kg)}{Height(metres) \times Height\ (metres)}$$

For example, somebody who weighs 65 kg and is 1.6 metres tall

BMI = 65 divided by (1.6 × 1.6)

BMI = 65 divided by 2.56

BMI = 25.4

If you are concerned about being overweight discuss this too with your therapist.

Some people anecdotally report that their emotions and mood are negatively affected by consuming foods that result in rapid increases in blood sugar followed by a rapid fall in blood sugar. These foods are referred to as high glycaemic index (GI) foods and include sugar and soft drinks. Others report an increase in agitation and anxiety after consuming caffeine-containing drinks an foods such as caffeine-containing cola drinks, energy drinks, and chocolate. It is pretty much standard for clinicians treating people with anxiety problems to recommend cutting back or stopping caffeine use as caffeine stimulates the system in the body associated with anxiety.

 Comment from Wendy

I often find at the end of the day that I am tired, and cooking a time-consuming nutritious meal is just too much. I combat this problem by planning at the beginning of each week so that I am sure that there is the right kind of food in the pantry that will support me eating nutritiously without having to do too much after a tough day. Planning also enables me to eat regular meals even when I am away from home

Exercise

We cannot recommend exercise *per se* for any single reader as we are not aware of your physical condition, what medications you are on, and whether you have any medical condition. However, we can discuss the concept of exercise in general.

Exercise has been shown to be beneficial in the treatment of anxiety and depression, as well as being excellent for our physical health. One of the hypotheses why exercise helps with depression is that exercise stimulates the release of our own 'feel good' chemicals called endorphins.

We all know that exercise is supposed to be good for us; however, unless we find the exercise sufficiently rewarding in either the short or long term we are unlikely to continue exercising. Struggling to maintain an exercise programme is not unique to people with BPD—most of the technologically developed world struggles with this.

Obviously exercise will only help if we do it! So the challenge is finding ways of exercising that we find satisfying enough. As with eating, the goal is to find a way of exercising that is sustainable for the rest of our lives. Start small and build up exercising in small steps. If you have any doubts as to your physical capacity to exercise, consult a physician.

Some people enjoy exercising by themselves, while others prefer exercising with others. An advantage of exercising with others is that we are more likely to exercise if we have made a commitment to another person. We are much less likely to be tempted to lie in bed on that cold morning if we have an exercise mate waiting at the end of the drive.

Some people like formal exercise programmes such as at gyms while others prefer informal exercise schedules. Having a regular time to exercise helps build exercise into our daily habits. Other practicalities are finding effective footwear if walking or running and exploring safe places to exercise.

If you can build in some reward/s that you can give yourself for developing healthy exercise patterns then do so. Do whatever you need to boost your desire, motivation, and commitment to sustainable exercise.

Alcohol and other non-prescribed mind–altering substances

Alcohol and other non-prescribed mind–altering drugs cloud our minds and can mess with our bodies. Using substances to block out emotional pain and distress is understandable if our lives are filled with pain and we are not aware of alternative healthier ways of coping. However, one of the problems with using substances as a solution to life's problems is that we avoid rather than solve problems and get no practice learning how to solve problems. There are alternative and healthier ways than using non-prescribed mind-altering substances to deal with distress. Learning these will also give us the skill for future problem solving. If you are using substances (alcohol and other drugs) as a way of getting by, discuss this with your therapist so that you can explore other healthier options.

Tending to medical and physical conditions

We need to be in the best possible shape we can be in to deal with what life throws at us. This includes ensuring that any medical or physical condition that we have is being optimally managed or treated. For example, any pain such as toothache will decrease our capacity to deal with the challenges of the day. If you take medication on an ongoing basis, make sure that you do not run out of medications. Tending to diabetes, asthma, and other medical illnesses will help maximize our emotional capacities. Eyesight, hearing, or joint problems that are well managed can improve our emotional resilience (hardiness).

40

Is it our relationship with something 'larger than ourselves' that makes a difference?

➔ Key points

◆ Research has shown that the majority of people believe in something 'larger than oneself' in a spiritual or religious sense. If you are one of this majority, it makes sense to attend to these areas of your life to achieve life balance and fulfilment.

◆ You can experience a sense of community in a wide range of ways such as belonging to local sports, book, singing, or music groups, or being part of the street or building you live in (greeting neighbours), or belonging to an AA, Narcotics Anonymous (NA), or other self-help group.

◆ We all value doing things that are meaningful even if they are not necessarily fun.

Research has shown that the majority of people believe in something 'larger than oneself' in a spiritual or religious sense. If you are one of this majority, it makes sense to attend to these areas of your life to achieve life balance and fulfilment.

Greater life fulfilment may result from a number of factors that range from lofty 'peak' experiences to pragmatic lifestyle behaviours (e.g. cigarettes, alcohol, street drugs). Other factors include awareness of the value of living in the present moment, experience of community, and the hope that comes from believing in something 'larger than oneself'. Prayer, meditation, contemplation, and mindfulness have been shown to be effective ways for relevant people to enhance their emotional well-being and lower their levels of stress.

If you are not a religious or spiritual person the news is still good. You can practise living in the present moment via attention control, contemplation, or mindfulness practice. You can experience a sense of community in a wide range of ways such as belonging to local sports, book, singing, or music groups, or being part of the street or building you live in (greeting neighbours), or belonging to an AA, Narcotics Anonymous (NA), GROW, or other self-help group. You can do something small for somebody else such as acknowledging and greeting a neighbour, smiling at the person delivering the mail, thanking the supermarket check-out operator, or enquiring after a friend's well-being.

We all value doing things that are meaningful even if they are not necessarily fun. For some of us this will involve the concept of 'service'. Examples may include visiting a sick friend, tending to children even though we are exhausted, feeding the dog, and going to vote on election day. We do these and other meaningful 'service' activities so that we live lives of integrity, in keeping with our important personal values and long-term visions for ourselves.

If you are an active participant in spiritual or religious life, you will know the avenues available to you. If you are interested in spiritual or religious life but not active, you could discuss with your therapist possible pathways to addressing this part of your life.

41

Notes to family and friends

> ## ➡ Key points
>
> ◆ We thank you for taking the time to read this book.
>
> ◆ We encourage you to learn what you can about the BPD condition.
>
> ◆ If you are a parent remember that your child may have been born with a biological vulnerability to intense emotional experiencing that was and is neither good nor bad but that nevertheless would have made it really hard for even the very best of parents and their child. In this situation nobody is to blame, neither the child nor the parent. Having this understanding can provide the necessary foundation for parents and their adult child to begin a process of healing.
>
> ◆ If you are realistic about the support you are able to offer, and the boundaries/limits you need to set, you are less likely to become exhausted and frustrated.
>
> ◆ There is very good reason to hope—people with BPD, on the whole, recover.

Thank you

Thank you for taking the time to read this book.

You and their struggles

When you are struggling with the enormous difficulty of supporting someone with BPD, it can be challenging to remember that the person that you care about or love is struggling too, in a battle with an intensity that feels to them akin to being in a combat zone. The very nature of the disorder means that relationships with others can be unstable, particularly with those they care most about and love the most. The person that you care about or love may do things that you find distressing, frustrating, or annoying. Generally the primary purpose of these behaviours is not to inflict pain upon you; rather they are often ineffective behaviours of a person trying to manage in a world they don't understand.

Knowledge

We encourage you to learn what you can about the BPD condition. We encourage you to be involved at the level that is right for you and to be completely open about your level of involvement.

Cause? One non—blaming understanding

If you are a parent remember that your child may have been born with a biological vulnerability to intense emotional experiencing that was and is neither good nor bad but that nevertheless would have made it really hard for even the very best of parents and their child. In this situation nobody is to blame, neither the child nor the parent. Having this understanding can provide the necessary foundation for parents and their adult child to begin a process of healing. You may wish to re-read Chapter 6 'What causes BPD?' in Section 1 of this book.

The long haul—limits/boundaries

It can be valuable for the person you care about or love for you to be around for the long haul. At times this might require setting limits or backing off somewhat to take some time for yourself. This is fine, and is likely to be the best thing you can do for the one you are supporting, if it is going to allow you to see the journey through in the long run. If you are realistic about the support you are able to offer, and the limits/boundaries you need to set, you are less likely to become exhausted and frustrated. It is generally most effective to be open and honest about your limits and boundaries, and to set these down at a time when everyone's emotional gauge is relatively low. Limits/boundaries set during a time of crisis are more likely to be experienced as punitive—it is far better to plan ahead, work out your limits, and make them clear to all—including the team treating the person you are supporting, if appropriate, ahead of time. If, during a time of turmoil, you feel the need to move your limits/boundaries, if at all possible wait until the crisis has passed and redefine the limits/boundaries when the emotional gauge is low again.

The person that you are supporting might want you involved in developing a plan for treatment with their therapist or treating team that is guided by their long-term goals. Being involved enables you to understand where the treatment is heading and the reasons behind various decisions, and also allows the support you are able to offer to be in the treatment plan as well as the limits of what you are able and willing to do. Sometimes treating clinicians make a decision with the person that you are supporting that the clinician/s will step back a little to encourage the person that you are supporting to try and manage crises using the skills they have developed or are developing. If you are not informed about and do not understand the rationale behind this, you might feel the urge to step in and help the person that you are supporting feel better—while feeling frustrated, hurt, and angry wondering why the therapist or treating team is not doing this. Not only is this exhausting for you, it could decrease opportunities for the person that you are supporting to learn how to manage the inevitable crises and challenges that life brings, in new ways. On the other hand, sometimes therapists or treating clinicians will want to be more active and involved than you feel is appropriate. If you are not informed about and do not agree with this stance, you could again feel frustrated, hurt, or angry, feeling that your efforts to help are being undermined. These scenarios indicate the value of having the person that you are supporting, treating clinicians, and yourself aligned regarding the directions of treatment wherever possible.

Communication

Be clear with your communications. When you love or care about someone with BPD, it can be tempting to avoid giving them information you would give others you are close to. We recommend an approach that recognizes that the person that you care about may be vulnerable but that you too have rights. What we mean by this is for you to be considered and compassionate in relating to the person that you care about, recognizing their vulnerability, but also to look after your life and yourself by not excessively tip-toeing around them.

Part of the person that you care about's journey is learning to live with the ups and downs that come as part of the human experience. Finding out after the event that information has been withheld from them may be more upsetting than having known at the earlier opportunity. The person that you care about needs to be able to practise their skills at times of upsetting news, such as a death or departure of someone important. Again we recommend a considered compassionate approach that recognizes their vulnerability and also treats them as an adult human being. These approaches are also more likely to decrease the need for you to be excessively and constantly guarded with what you are saying in front of them.

Skills

As part of the person you care about's journey to recovery, they will be learning new skills to deal with the emotions they experience, and the world in general. One of the things you can do as a support person is learn those skills alongside them, and encourage use of the skills being learnt at appropriate times. You may be pleasantly surprised as often the skills the person you care about is learning will be things that we can all utilize in our day-to-day lives.

Family/friends groups

Some regions have groups for family and friends of people with BPD. These groups vary from an informal support group to structured groups offering skills training. Sharing your journey with others can be of great benefit both to you and to others in the group, and sometimes is one of the few places where others understand the journey you are travelling. On the other hand, it is possible that you find such meetings lead to a lot more distress than you feel able to handle effectively. If you attend such a group, assess the advantages and disadvantages of your attending and feel that you have a right to engage at a level that is right for you—that is, a level that is going to be most effective.

Safety

Where safety issues are present, we encourage you to share this with professional/s.

Guideline list

Below we outline some guidelines for family members that have been cited by Gunderson (2001) and Friedel (2004) in separate books and on Dr Friedel's website. The guidelines apply equally well to friends and other support people. These guidelines headings are offered to provide some structure for you to think about how to go about matters and in no way do we wish glibly to imply that carrying out the guidelines is an easy task. Further information on Friedel's guidelines can easily be obtained on his website if you have internet access.

Solve big problems in small steps
Keep things 'cool'
Maintain family routines
Listen
Collaborate and be consistent
Limit setting: be direct but careful

Gunderson (2001)

Learn about the disorder
Seek professional help (Friedel suggests helping the person with BPD access help if necessary)
Support the treatment programme
Attempt to remain calm
Respond consistently to problematic behaviours
Participate in educational experiences about borderline disorder
Remember: the person with BPD must take charge
Join a borderline disorder consumer and family support organization (Friedel names NEA-BPD and NAMI as organizations to approach for this information)
Remain positive and optimistic
Take good care of yourself

Friedel (2004; bpddemystified.com)

Hope

As a final word to family and friends; have hope. There is very good reason to hope—people with BPD on the whole recover. You may like to glance back to the chapters in this book on prognosis and treatment effectiveness, and remind yourself that life improves for the majority of people with the condition—and sometimes you may need to carry that hope when the person you care about is not able to.

Thank you

Thank you for taking the time to read this chapter/book and if you choose to do so, for sharing and supporting the person that you care about or love through their journey of exploring pathways to healing and recovery

References for family and friends

Bochain NR, Porr V, Villagran NE, (2002). *New hope for people with borderline personality disorder*. New York: Three Rivers Press.

Friedel RO (2004). *Borderline personality disorder demystified: an essential guide for understanding and living with BPD.* New York: Marlowe, pp. 190–196. (Dr Friedel's website at time of writing in 2007: www.bpddemystified.com)

Gunderson JG, Hoffman PD (eds) (2005). *Understanding and treating borderline personality disorder: a guide for professionals and families.* Washington DC: American Psychiatric Publishing.

42

Concluding comments to the reader

 Comment from Wendy

Have hope.

I was once considered a hopeless case and am now working, and leading an active social life. My journey of recovery has been like climbing a mountain. As I climbed higher, I discovered I was a strong, capable, and likeable woman. I have not reached all my goals yet but now mostly enjoy the journey I walk. I am now genuinely living a life with long-term goals and a vision for the future; something I didn't have before and didn't think was possible.

Writing this book has been a powerful and moving experience, requiring as it did considerable emotional reflection on my life—past, present, and future. I have shared with you all the skills I learned on my journey, attempting to combine these into a meaningful whole.

All our journeys of recovery will be different; however, my wish is that your journey will have been made a little easier for having read something in this book that will make a positive difference for you.

Thank you for reading parts or all of this book. It has been a real pleasure for

> **Explore how you can take charge of your recovery**

us to write the book and we hope it has been of benefit for you. If the book has been helpful by enabling you to move forward just one step in your recovery, it will have been worth the effort.

We leave you with our single most important communication,

We wish you the very best in your journey to recovery and in your life beyond recovery.

Glossary

Affect—A description of one's mood or emotion at a specific moment in time

Agoraphobia—DSM-IV diagnosis. Anxiety, usually about being in unfamiliar situations

Alcohol and other substance dependence or abuse—DSM-IV diagnosis. Physical dependence or problems related to alcohol or substance use

Binge eating disorder—Proposal for DSM V diagnosis. Binge eating without 'inappropriate' (sic) behaviours preventing weight gain such as fasting, vomiting, purgative/laxative usage, and excess exercise (see Bulimia for comparison)

Bipolar disorder/bipolar affective disorder—DSM-IV diagnosis—a condition typically characterized by episodes of depression and mania (excessively elevated or irritable mood, racy thoughts, and other features requiring hospitalization)

Bipolar II disorder—DSM-IV diagnosis—a condition with episodes of depression and hypomania (features like those of mania but are of shorter duration or do not result in hospitalization)

Bulimia—DSM-IV diagnosis. Binge eating associated with 'inappropriate' (sic) behaviours preventing weight gain such as fasting, vomiting, purgative/laxative usage, and excess exercise

Controlled trial—a scientific study where one group receive one treatment and another group receive a different treatment

DBT—Dialectical behaviour therapy. Behaviour therapy plus acceptance and mindfulness practices of Eastern meditation traditions

Depressive disorder—DSM-IV diagnosis. Usually refers to being depressed for a discrete time period

Diagnostic and Statistical Manual of Mental Disorders fourth edition This manual is the major diagnostic reference for professionals, outlining features required for a diagnosis to be made in accordance with the DSM-IV manual.

Dysthymic disorder—DSM-IV diagnosis. Refers to being depressed for long periods (more than 2 years) at a lower level usually than with a depressive disorder

Generalized anxiety disorder—DSM-IV diagnosis. Anxiety in many areas of life

Mentalizing/mentalization—the capacity to observe, reflect—and seek to understand mental states and how these arise

Neurotic—A term no longer in regular use. Used to refer to people who had distressing difficulties in relationship with themselves or others

Obsessive-compulsive disorder—DSM-IV diagnosis. Anxiety due to intrusive irrational thoughts that the person recognizes as their own followed by a 'compulsion' activity that serves to decrease the anxiety although the activity is recognized as irrational. For example, irrational fears of germs resulting in hand washing

Panic disorder—DSM-IV diagnosis. Discrete (usually less than 30 minutes) overwhelming episodes of anxiety

Post-traumatic stress disorder—DSM-IV diagnosis. Anxiety clearly linked with a psychological trauma, often with invasive memories of the trauma and an excessively high level of general vigilance (watchfulness) and alertness

Prognosis—A scientific prediction of the statistical likelihood of certain outcomes

Psychodynamic therapy—a therapy where the relationship between therapist and client is seen as the central and most important factor in achieving change

Psychoanalytical therapy—same as psychodynamic therapy but more pure in approach

Psychotic—a condition typically associated with delusions (fixed false belief) and/or hallucinations (false perceptions, e.g. hearing voice of person who is not present)

Randomized controlled trial—a scientific study where clients are randomly allocated to two or more groups, with one group receiving one treatment and the other group/s receive a different treatment. This is a higher scientific standard than a controlled trial.

Social phobia—DSM-IV diagnosis. Anxiety about social situations usually with avoidance of social situations

Schizophrenia—DSM-IV diagnosis—a condition typically associated with episodes of psychosis and other features

Schema—a deep core belief system that might be helpful, ineffective, or harmful

Traits—some features or characteristics of

Uncontrolled trial—a scientific study where clients outcomes are measured comparing how they are after treatment with how they were before treatment. This is a lower level of scientific standard than a controlled trial or randomized controlled trial.

References

References

American Psychiatric Association (2000). *Diagnostic and statistical manual of mental disorders*, 4th edn. Text Revision. Washington DC: American Psychiatric Association.

Bartels N, Crotty T (1998). *A systems approach to treatment: the borderline personality disorder skill training manual*. Winfield IL: EID Treatment Systems.

Beck A, Freeman A, Pretzer J, Davis DD, Fleming B, Ottaviani R, Beck J, Simon KM, Padesky C, Meyer J, Trexler L (1990). *Cognitive therapy of personality disorders*. New York: Guilford Press, pp. 186–187.

Clarke D (2003). Faith and hope. *Australasian Psychiatry* **11**: 164–168.

Desmond L (2004). Life on the borderline. *A Life in the Day* **8**(2): 4–7.

Friedel RO (2004). *Borderline personality disorder demystified: an essential guide for understanding and living with BPD*. New York: Marlowe, pp. 190–196. (Dr Friedel's website at time of writing in 2007: www.bpddemystified.com)

Gunderson JG (2001). Family therapies. 9. In: *Borderline personality disorder: a clinical guide*. Washington: American Psychiatric Publishing, p. 204.

Joyce PR, McKenzie JM, Mulder RT, Luty SE, Sullivan PF, Miller AL, Kennedy MA (2006). Genetic, developmental and personality correlates of self-mutilation in depressed patients. *Australian and New Zealand Journal of Psychiatry* **40**: 225–229.

Krawitz R, Watson C (2003). *Borderline personality disorder: a practical guide to treatment*. Oxford: Oxford University Press.

Kreisman JJ, Straus H (1991). *I hate you, don't leave me*. New York: Avon Press.

Linehan MM (1993a). *Cognitive-behavioral therapy treatment of borderline personality disorder*. New York: Guilford Press.

Linehan MM (1993b). *Skills training manual for treating borderline personality disorder*. New York: Guilford Press.

Linehan MM, (2003). *From suffering to freedom: practicing reality acceptance*. From Chaos to Freedom Video Series. Behavioral Tech LLC.

Miller WR, Rollnick S (2002). *Motivational interviewing*. New York: Guilford Press.

Milton I, Banfai A (1999). Basic principles for understanding severe personality disorder. 1. In: *Guidelines for working with serious personality disorder* (Milton I, McMahon K, eds). Melbourne: Psychoz, pp. 1–7.

Prochaska JO, Norcross JC, Diclemente CC (1994). *Changing for good.* New York: Harper Collins.

Torgerson S, Lygren S, Oien PA, Skre I, Onstad S, Edvardsen J, Tambs K, Kringlen E (2000). A twin study of personality disorders. *Comprehensive Psychiatry* 41: 416–425.

Whitfield CL (1993). *Boundaries and relationships: knowing enjoying and protecting the self.* Deerfield Beach: Health Communications.

Zanarini MC, Frankenburg FR, Dubo ED (1998). Axis II comorbidity of borderline personality disorder. *Comprehensive Psychiatry* 39: 296–302.

Zanarini MC, Frankenburg FR, Hennen J, Reich D, Silk KR (2004a). Axis I comorbidity in patients with borderline personality disorder: 6-year follow-up and prediction of time to remission. *American Journal of Psychiatry* 161: 2108–2114.

Zanarini MC, Frankenburg FR, Vujanovic AA, Hennen J, Reich D, Silk KR (2004b). Axis II comorbidity in patients with borderline personality disorder: 6-year follow-up and prediction of time to remission. *American Journal of Psychiatry* 110: 416–420.

Zanarini MC, Frankenburg FR, Hennen J, Reich D, Silk KR (2005). The Mclean study of adult development (MSAD): overview and implications of the first six years of prospective follow-up. *International Journal of Personality Disorder* 19: 505–523.

Zanarini MC, Frankenburg FR, Hennen J, Reich DB, Silk KR (2006). Prediction of the 10-year course of borderline personality disorder. *American Journal of Psychiatry* 163: 827–832.

Index